Jennifer has once again wri
any other that will jumpst
I have personally observe
even on several international trips for nine days
and friends, and she is the real deal. Don't walk, but run to read
this book. Its cutting-edge recipes will change your health and
add quality years to your life as you look and feel amazing.

—Dr. David Herzog
Author, *Jumpstart!*

Jennifer's creativity shines through with raw and healthy recipes
to tantalize your taste buds and tempt your tummy. This book is
a must-have, go-to resource for anyone serious about detoxifying
in a healthy and holistic way. It is an intelligently written, fun,
and inspiring culinary resource to maximize your good health.

—Susan Kleinschmidt
CEO, Good Insights Strategy

Jennifer has a passion for food and healthy living and it is so evident in how she lives out her life. I'm certain that whoever reads
this book will benefit greatly in improving their lifestyle.

—Gary Lim
CEO, North America Flagship Food Group

Original and practical, simple yet comprehensive, Jennifer Mac's
first-hand account of zestfully eating one's way back to health is
a gift to all who want to nourish both their health and eating
pleasure.

—David McCown
Owner, Treasure Valley Salsa

As an active seventy-seven-year-old video journalist working on
numerous dangerous assignments, I find it necessary to keep
my body and mind as physically fit as possible. Jennifer's book
is a carefully researched work, providing delicious and nutritionally advanced recipes to help lose weight, restore proper body

functions, and give us the vitality that God intended for us to have.

—Patrick Matrisciana
Founder, Jeremiah Films

We at *Global Gourmet Magazine* congratulate Jennifer Mac for her new book, *Detox Delish*. The book will surely benefit the lives of many people, just as Jennifer's regular column in our publication has been enhancing the health and lifestyle of our readers all over. *Detox Delish* truly embraces the natural goodness of foods for wellness and vitality, offering wise and wide approaches to creative flavors enjoyable by palates of all cultures.

—Ricky Xu
Publisher, *Global Gourmet Magazine*

An honest, pure, and informative book straight from the heart. Jennifer has a beautiful way of blending her recipes into her personal life instances. *Detox Delish* is a clear example of "practice before you preach," and Jennifer has kept it simple and doable. A warm and refreshing book which is a must-have for everyone and I will definitely share with many of my personal and professional friends.

—Vijaykumar Mirchandani
Award-winning Documentary Filmmaker, *Where The Streets Have No Name* and *They Are No Less*

Detox Delish

Jennifer Mac

SILOAM

Most CHARISMA HOUSE BOOK GROUP products are available at special quantity discounts for bulk purchase for sales promotions, premiums, fund-raising, and educational needs. For details, write Charisma House Book Group, 600 Rinehart Road, Lake Mary, Florida 32746, or telephone (407) 333-0600.

DETOX DELISH by Jennifer Mac
Published by Siloam
Charisma Media/Charisma House Book Group
600 Rinehart Road
Lake Mary, Florida 32746
www.charismahouse.com

Cover design by Vincent Pirozzi
Cover photo by Tana Photography
Design Director: Justin Evans

Visit the author's website at TheJenniferMac.com.

Library of Congress Cataloging-in-Publication Data
Names: Mac, Jennifer, author.
Title: Detox delish / Jennifer Mac.

Description: First edition. | Lake Mary, Florida : Siloam, [2016]
Identifiers: LCCN 2016045381| ISBN 9781629989105 (trade
paper) | ISBN 9781629989112 (ebook)
Subjects: LCSH: Detoxification (Health)
Classification: LCC RA784.5 .M28 2016 | DDC 613.2--dc23
LC record available at https://lccn.loc.gov/2016045381

First edition

16 17 18 19 20 — 987654321
Printed in the United States of America

To Dad and Mom, thank you for your encouragement and support.

Thank you, God, for Your guidance, love, and peace on this amazing, destiny-filled, and unexpected journey.

Contents

RECIPES

Acknowledgments

To Dr. Huber, thank you for the time you spent with me and for your tireless efforts and research to educate the public on the struggle to keep our food supply safe for future generations. Both you and my dad, a conventional farmer who turned radical evangelist on the importance and sustainability of soil health, have taught me that the best food begins with living, nutrient-dense soil. Thank you to my friend, Gloria Westerfield, for reviewing one of my first drafts and for your prayers.

To Maureen Eha, thank you for your oversight, guidance, and input throughout this book project. To Marcos Perez, Joshua Dorlon, Althea Thompson, and Margarita Henry, thank you for your marketing expertise and invaluable guidance—I'm so appreciative. To Megan Turner, Leigh DeVore, Deborah Moss, Kimberly Overcast, and Anne Mulchan, thank you for your reviews, edits, and feedback. Your attention to detail is valued and did not go unnoticed. To Tessie DeVore, thank you for taking the chance on a farm girl's dream to write some healthy recipes. I also want to thank Cheria Soria and the family at Living Light Culinary Institute.

Foreword

*I*FIRST HEARD ABOUT Jennifer through her father, George, while we were both giving talks on fermented foods. The next day I met her mother, Carol, and she introduced me to Jennifer's first book, *The Right Blend: Blender-Only Raw Food Recipes*. I had been studying foods as healing agents for some time and was familiar with the benefit of eating raw foods (they have the highest enzyme contents). I always ate a lot of salads and drank juices and smoothies but had not yet ventured into the world of completely raw foods. Flipping through Jennifer's book, I was amazed at the recipes and wanted to taste as many dishes as possible. My husband's birthday was just around the corner, and I decided to give him a birthday party quite different from the usual. I contacted Jennifer about serving mostly raw foods, including his birthday cake. I did not tell him what I was serving at the party except that I was hiring a chef because, if he knew, I would have certainly met strong resistance.

Jennifer and I planned ahead and decided on foods from her book. The guests were all amazed that raw foods were very tasty—for most of them, this was their first exposure to a completely raw, mostly vegan dinner, including a birthday cheesecake with raspberry topping. The delicious foods helped make for a special evening.

This book, *Detox Delish*, is about cleansing and detoxification with many delicious recipes that I have been waiting for. I left the standard American diet (SAD) and the modern American diet (MAD) years ago. I have become gluten free and bovine milk free except for butter, ghee, and cream. I recently added fermented foods to my diet, a topic Jennifer speaks extensively about in the book. Jennifer's guidance and knowledge is now taking me into the world of raw and whole-food detox foods that I will incorporate into my eating regimen.

I have been practicing neurology since 1982. Like any other conventional physician, I pursued drug treatments for most of the neurological ailments, including epilepsy, headaches, multiple sclerosis, neuropathy, Parkinson's disease, and Alzheimer's disease. I saw promised medications come and go and came to realize that, though they do have a place in my practice, they were never the sole answer to the problems. It is similar to other physical disorders. For instance, we cannot cure hypertension even with so many high blood pressure medications available. However, when patients lose weight (if needed), eat more nourishing foods, drink more water, and exercise, generally their blood pressure naturally drops to a normal level for that person. I began wondering if neurological problems could be helped by changes in lifestyle and diet as well. What I have been witnessing has been just amazing. When patients are given directions and knowledge in the areas of exercise, hydration, healthy eating, and more, they figure things out. All they needed was the confirmation that they are on the right path to health. Often patients can reduce the medications and, if it is their goal, eventually come off them safely.

The first step for these patients is to detox from the SAD and MAD regimens they have been on for years. Jennifer's new book is a very valuable addition to my armamentarium and will be the first on the list of the references I give to my patients. I hope it is yours too.

—Mihoko Nelsen, MD
Neurologist

Introduction

*H*AVE YOU EVER considered yourself a victim of groupthink, the tendency to follow the popular thoughts and beliefs within the group? Have you ever questioned life, your surroundings, or even your health? I did. I had to. I'll never forget when the doctor said I'd be on medication for the rest of my life. He explained that diseases are degenerative and my medication would only increase with age. This was my fate, or so I thought. I entered my late teens and twenties feeling fatigued, bloated, and clouded in my thinking. For over ten years I was on medication for Hashimoto's thyroiditis, a form of hypothyroidism—otherwise known as an underactive thyroid. While the story ends well, my path to health and wholeness was indirect, zigzagged, and nothing short of an international and culinary adventure.

Propaganda

Kale me crazy, but fruit slices and leafy greens must no longer be subjected to mere garnishes for SAD (Standard American Diet) plates or fluffy bedding to make salad bars look pretty. Please *lettuce* tell you the hardcore *flax*: in order to leave SAD meals behind, our bodies need to be cleansed from the unfruitful habits (pun intended) of processed sugars, white flours, and fried oils. One way to transition out of SAD is to eat raw foods—juiced, blended, and eaten whole. Some dismiss this information as a *conspi-raw-cy*, just to get out of eating more veggies.

You do not have to eat one hundred percent raw, vegetarian, or vegan to benefit from the plant-based, *raw-some* recipes in this book. With obesity, diabetes, heart disease, and cancer at all-time highs, I'm asking you to depart from the SAD state of normal and enter the path to the *pa-raw-normal*. No pressure to join a *raw-volution* here. Instead, *beet* the system by putting an end to dieting and calorie counting, and start eating real, whole foods that satisfy the appetite and nourish every organ and cell.

As the body pushes the junk out of the trunk, you may encounter bursts of energy as well as phases of fatigue through this cleansing process known as detoxification. As you turn the pages of this book you may undergo *reprog-raw-mming*, loving the delicious ways fruits, vegetables, nuts, seeds, and sprouts can be prepared. You will be amazed at the vibrant flavors of creation's produce, not to mention the nutrient-rich, power-packed satisfaction real food provides. *Orange* you curious how a detoxed lifestyle can change your life? Join me on this journey to be deliciously healthy.

FRESH OFF THE FARM

Growing up on a vegetable farm in Idaho, fresh air, clean water, and seasonal produce surrounded me. My dad used to own an apple orchard in Washington years ago, so our home in Idaho was surrounded by trees he planted that produced mouthwatering stone fruits. The town was Fruitland. With a name like that, no wonder the peaches were sweeter, the plums juicier, and the apples crispier than any from supermarkets. For summer projects I grew gardens. I was the novice, but it was my grandparents who were master gardeners. My Japanese American grandfather and grand-mother *each* grew gardens on separate plots of land. Abundant were raspberries, strawberries, cucumbers, sweet corn, tomatoes, and melons—too much produce to name here.

In high school FFA (previously known as Future Farmers of America), like a scene straight out of *Napoleon Dynamite*, I was in the milk and cheese judging contest for the state of Idaho. In my spare time I studied weeds for the state's weed identification contest. I went on to compete nationally in farm business management. Farm life was part of the benefits package that came with country living. Few Americans have the opportunity to grow up on a farm, which was something I could not genuinely appreciate until years later when I lived and worked in cities with skylines and subway systems.

MY HEALTH

I was born with a ventricular septal defect, a hole in the wall dividing the left and right ventricles of my heart, otherwise known as a heart murmur. Thankfully this condition never limited me from having a normal life or playing sports. In fact, I never viewed myself as ill. At an attempt at eating healthy, I preferred bottled juice over soda pop and chose whole wheat bread over white. Nevertheless, even with a love for fruit and vegetables, my idea of a healthy meal was just *adding* them in, like a small bowl of fruit or a side salad.

The truth is I ate many over-processed and additive-filled foods from cans, packages, and boxes labeled "healthy," "low fat," or "low calorie." Most of the foods I ate were fried, zapped, and coated with chemicals. Little did I know destroying the nutrients was destroying me. Despite my efforts my diet too closely resembled the standard American diet. Being health conscious and being healthy are not synonymous, and good intentions can lead to deadly consequences.

During high school I felt sluggish and tired. Friends would tease me about falling asleep during movies. I continuously felt bloated, which I know now was inflammation due to toxicity. Later, during my undergraduate studies, I once visited the campus clinic about feeling so run-down. Not knowing that most doctors do not like patients diagnosing themselves, I shared my suspicion of a nutrient deficiency as a cause for my fatigue. After all, my grandmother's advice to eat more fresh fruits and vegetables always echoed in my mind. At the clinic I was assured this was not the case. What did I learn that day? I was told that the most basic box of dry cereal flakes is complete with all the nutrients a person needs to function—something I later learned to be false. I should have stuck to my grandmother's advice.

A few years later my friend Cathy suggested my symptoms sounded like a thyroid disorder, so I headed to a medical clinic. Not learning my first lesson of doctor-patient protocol, I extended my concern of a looming problem with my thyroid, placing my hands over my throat for a dramatic visual. The doctor assured me that was not the case. I insisted on a blood test, and was given a *simple* blood test, which came back normal.

The walk from the clinic to the car was one of defeat. A twenty-something-year-old should be at the top of her prime, but that wasn't me. Were all these symptoms in my head? A small light of hope rose up in me, and before driving away I knew I needed to get a second opinion. I'm grateful to this day for the doctor who gave me a second opinion and recognized a goiter—an enlarged thyroid—that was three to four times the normal size. The doctor performed a blood test that came back pointing to Hashimoto's disease.

On one hand, I was upset, because who wants to be associated with having a disease? On the other hand, it was a relief to put a name alongside the symptoms. Once on medication I started to feel better. However, I still didn't feel great. Some years later I found a piece of paper with symptoms I jotted down to share with an endocrinologist. On the worn out, crumpled old note was scribbled:

- Fatigue

- Long sleep

- Need naps

- Sluggish

- Bloated

- Constipated

- Slow-thinking

- Cold extremities

- Dazed and foggy

- Mood swings

- Loss of hair

- Dry and flaky skin

- Imbalanced

I once ran a marathon and decided walking wasn't an option. Unfortunately I got lost after mile marker twenty-four by following a group of runners down the wrong trail. Confused and disappointed, I turned around and kept running—a feeble hobble resembling running—until I eventually reached the finish line. With this same spirit of determination, I combed through materials and books seeking ways to improve my health.

As an optimist who needed answers, I wasn't about to give up. Over the first few years I transitioned to eating more whole foods, such as cooked vegetables and whole seeds, grains, and legumes, acquainting myself with different foods, such as mung beans, flaxseed oil, and spirulina. In 2001 and 2002 I was working in Boise, Idaho. I had read that cold-pressed coconut oil was good for thyroid function, and I found a couple stores that carried it. Today it is a must-have staple in my kitchen, but at the time I had no idea how to use it in its raw form. As I did with flaxseed oil, I'd take a spoonful or two at a time. I was getting better, but it would still take a few more years before I was able to get off medication completely and be disease free.

WORLDVIEW IN RECOVERY

I have lived in Seoul, Hong Kong, Chengdu, Shanghai, and Beijing, to name a few places. What started out as university exchange programs transitioned to work and business opportunities. These same opportunities furthered my journey of health and wholeness. On a semester exchange program in Seoul, I ate high amounts of vegetable-based dishes. Fermented foods are abundant in Korea. Sometimes I ate kimchee, a spicy fermented cabbage (recipe in chapter 9), three times a day. It was in Korea that I started to feel lighter, less inflamed, and less constipated. I attribute this to the large amounts of fermented vegetables I was eating. (See more about fermentation and probiotics in chapter 5.)

After my stints in Asia I moved back to Idaho, entered graduate school, and worked in international business for the departments of agriculture and commerce with responsibilities over Asia. After finishing my graduate studies, I returned to China to further my language studies and find work in business. Living in Asia, I could not help but see the world differently, including how I viewed food and health. A Chinese friend compared my Western view to her Chinese view of health through the analogy of a boiling pot, with the heat representing disease. The Western approach in cooling the pot was to throw ice cubes into the pot. The Chinese approach, in contrast, was to slowly turn down the temperature of the burner. It is clear now that the medication I was on was not curing my disease; it was only treating the symptoms. I was taught that my condition was permanent and all I had to do was take pills. However, my experiences kept challenging this belief. An American friend, a doctor of veterinary medicine, once noticed during surgeries on dogs that sometimes their thyroid problems would disappear. During my time studying in China, I shared my thyroid disorder with a fellow student. She, in turn, shared her own experience of having a goiter, an inflamed thyroid gland, around the age of five or six. Her mother, having connections with a local hospital, obtained human placenta to feed her for its healing properties and high mineral content. My friend was then fed bowlfuls of seaweed for its high mineral content, especially iodine. I listened to this story with one thing staring me in the face: she no longer had a goiter. It was gone.

Ready for some real changes in my health, I gave seaweed a try. At the university in China it was a common dish in the cafeteria, and we paid for it by weight. It is a good thing I loved sea vegetables, because I ate a lot—spaghetti serving-size amounts, in fact, for about three months. This led to my first detoxification experience. Sea vegetables not only provide perhaps the richest source of minerals, but they also chelate heavy metals and other toxins out of the system. The main raw food I was eating during this period was fresh melon in the morning as an antidote to keep from feeling constipated. Now on seaweed as well, my body started eliminating more times per day than the number of meals I was eating. This newfound digestion surprised me. Shortly after beginning this diet and beginning to practice *wushu*, a Chinese martial art, I noticed sensations of lightness, agility, and more energy. The mental and physical cloudiness and fogginess started to lift. My hair, that had been breaking off almost continuously, became thicker and fuller.

During a trip home I saw my endocrinologist. My thyroid medication kept being lowered, and this time she asked me what I was doing. There was a laundry list of things I told her, from vitamin supplements to medicinal herbs to flaxseed oil to seaweed. Jotting down my list of remedies and still looking down, she said, "Don't eat too much." It occurred to me that the seaweed could alter my medication, and since I was on such a low dose it could mean tipping me over the edge—possibly allowing me to become medication free. I share this with you not to point to one miracle food as the cure-all. This is my personal experience. I now eat seaweed in small amounts, such as snacking on a nori seaweed sheet, mixing in kombu in soups, or sprinkling dulse on salads. They have a wonderful savory quality and are one of the richest sources of minerals around.

In 2007 I transitioned to a diet high in raw foods. This was another factor contributing to the detoxification and healing my body experienced. The raw foods I was eating replaced many health-destroying foods, such as refined flours, refined sugars, and genetically engineered (GE) foods containing genetically modified organisms (GMOs). Most of the GE food staples available today are not eaten in their uncooked, raw form so my eating mostly raw foods automatically eliminated many of these foods.

Do I believe eating raw food to be the cure for all ailments? No. But I'm convinced that eating raw food played a critical role in my detoxification and recovery. Many people assume I am a raw vegan due to my culinary background. Today my diet is primarily plant-based, with a big supply of fresh and raw foods. However, I do not adhere to one particular diet or eating regimen. It seems like there's a new one every year, right? When I was growing up, my family ate a lot of produce from the farm and garden, and my dad bought cow's and goat's milk from the locals. Hence, my plant-based diet occasionally includes grass-fed animal products. A couple of my favorites are organic, free-range eggs from the family farm and probiotic, organic kefir.

Many of my clients are vegan or adhere to strict food preferences and guidelines. How my clients choose to eat is a personal—and respected—choice. I work with all kinds of food and diet preferences, food intolerances, and doctor-prescribed restrictions.

Despite one's diet, chances are one commonality is the need for more fresh, plant-based produce. Eating raw provides the highest amount of vitamins, micronutrients, phytonutrients, and enzymes possible. It's simple: eating raw gives you the most bang for your bite.

As Hippocrates said, "Let food be thy medicine and medicine be thy food."[1]

Over the years my mind-set completely changed on how I thought of health and wholeness.

Old mind-set

These words and phrases were the focus of my mind before my mind-set changed:

- Slimming
- Weight control
- Quick fix
- Fat free
- Calorie burning
- Low sugar
- Low calories
- Low carb
- Diet food
- Meat equals protein

My new mind-set on food

These words and phrases are the focus of my mind now:

- Transformed
- Cleansing
- Longevity
- Chemical free
- Energy providing
- Natural sugars
- Nutrient dense
- Living foods
- Beautifying foods
- GMO free

Detox Delish

If you have opened my book and read this far, there is a chance you are searching for a change in your life. Perhaps your doctor put you on a detox program, and you are in need of recipes. Maybe you discovered gluten and dairy products are off limits and now you are desperate for more options. Or you may be a health-conscious individual looking to maximize your range of nutritionally packed recipes for everyday living. Whether you are any of the above or simply curious, I'm so excited to share my passion of health, wholeness, and delicious recipes with you!

CHAPTER 1

Green It Like You Mean It

A CHILDHOOD FRIEND ONCE commented that if she were an animal, she would be a horse because they were so beautiful and lean. She had a point. I contemplated why most humans didn't compare to the beauty and strength of horses with their luminous and shiny coats of hair and muscular and curved physical builds. Growing up in the country, I saw cows and horses graze on green grasses in fields all day long. During the cold months, they ate dried alfalfa and licked blocks of mineral and salt. However, much of their diet consisted of fresh vegetation. What if I ate the same way and switched to eating grass, or raw vegetables, all day? Contemplation soon turned into rationalization. After all, I was human. One could almost feel sorry for the species not benefiting from the modern conveniences of microwaves, can openers, and fast food. I dismissed the notion of eating a diet high in raw foods as unrealistic. That is, until a few years later.

I was in a bit of amazement when I encountered my first group of raw food eaters while I was studying at Living Light Culinary Institute in Northern California. People from all over the world come there to learn the art of raw vegan cuisine. At the time I was two years into eating a high raw diet while based overseas in Beijing, China, where I studied Mandarin Chinese and worked in the city's famous pearl market district. As the only American girl doing business inside the market, both Chinese and foreigners did double takes when they saw, behind the counter, an American girl staring back at them. Obviously I am not one to shy away from unconventional paths, so starting to *uncook* with raw foods, and to become a whole foods and raw food chef later, seemed just another anomaly on the road less traveled.

Class began every morning at the institute with a green smoothie breakfast bar. New to green smoothies, I quickly poured myself a glass, sat down, and observed these green smoothie veterans. Up until this time I had been eating raw foods in the forms of trail mix, apples, pears, bananas, carrots, and celery.

Looking at those around me, from the students to the staff, it was hard not to notice how amazing some of these people looked. Some appeared ten to fifteen years younger than their age. I was confronted with people in their forties, fifties, and sixties who were in excellent health and ate a diet similar to those animals grazing in the fields. Even those over sixty had a natural glow others their age, or younger, lacked. They seemed confident—and almost arrogant—carrying around glass jars of green concoctions consisting of blended leafy greens and fruits. It became evident that a common denominator in their eating regimen was the high amount of micronutrient-packed and chlorophyll-rich leafy greens and vitamin-bursting and fibrous fruits.

FOOD FOR THOUGHT: PLANT-BASED DOESN'T NECESSARILY MEAN VEGAN

When I tell people I teach raw food cuisine, they often ask two questions: "Are you a vegan?" asking if I eat no meat, dairy, or animal by-products, and "Do you eat only raw food?" I admit I'm not big on titles. I once read someone claim to be one hundred percent vegan ninety-nine percent of the time. Often titles serve as standards of how we see ourselves and the ideals of how we like others to see us. Some of my classmates were vegans, consuming no animal or honeybee products. Others incorporated raw animal products, such as raw fish, raw honey, and raw, unpasteurized dairy into their diets. Because my diet is primarily plant-based, most of my meals fall under the category of vegan, but I am not vegetarian or vegan.

Most define their diet (vegan, vegetarian, or some form of intolerance) by what they *do not* eat. My personal philosophy on food is that it is not so much of what we don't eat, but rather what we *do* eat. The Bible says: "Then God said, 'See, I have given you every plant yielding seed which is on the face of all the earth, and every tree which has fruit yielding seed. It shall be food for you'" (Gen. 1:29). This passage is often quoted to promote a vegan diet. I believe this passage is promoting a plant-based diet. However, I do not interpret this passage to be promoting strictly a vegan diet necessarily.

The Daniel fast of eating vegetables and water is often used to promote a vegan lifestyle. While Daniel went for periods of time on plant foods, whether on a fast or otherwise, Daniel's lifestyle was one of eating a clean, plant-based diet, but he was not vegan throughout his entire life. Later the Book of Daniel records that Daniel went on another fast, eating "no tasty food, no meat or wine" to mourn over a disturbing vision he was shown of future events to come (Dan. 10:3). Abstaining from meat for a period of time implies Daniel was not always eating a vegan diet, but it is implied that he was conscientious about what he put in his body.

Other verses in the Bible pertaining to the food we eat are listed here:

- "Every moving thing that lives will be food for you. I give you everything, just as I gave you the green plant" (Gen. 9:3). God gave us animals to eat, but it's also safe to say that God's original diet before the fall of man was the Genesis 1:29 diet—just plant-based.

- "'All things are lawful to me,' but not all things are helpful" (1 Cor. 6:12). When I began teaching raw food classes, many in my church circles were excited about my renewed health. However, I heard some insinuations that teaching on something as strict as a raw-ingredient recipe may be leaning on the side of legalism. After all, who wants to be deceived, especially if it tastes like sawdust? If only they knew how delicious health can be.

- "For the drunkard and the glutton will come to poverty" (Prov. 23:21). I believe Christians, especially in America, simply do not want to give up this one last indulgence—gluttony. Quit smoking? Check. Quick drinking? Check. Give up SAD food? No way! But what if a diet change wasn't birthed out of legalism? What if the foods God created, in their original and natural form, were the most delicious foods around? Health may begin to taste so delicious that you'll forget you were even being disciplined!

- "What? Do you not know that your body is the temple of the Holy Spirit, who is in you, whom you have received from God, and that you are not your own? You were bought with a price. Therefore glorify God in your body and in your spirit, which are God's" (1 Cor. 6:19–20). It is important to honor God with our physical bodies, not just in spirit.

- "Beloved, I pray that all may go well with you and that you may be in good health, even as your soul is well" (1 John 3:2). Personally, I cannot think of a better witness than for our spiritual health to parallel our physical and mental health.

- "Do you not know that you are the temple of God, and that the Spirit of God dwells in you? If anyone defiles the temple of God, God will destroy him. For the temple of God is holy. And you are His temple" (1 Cor. 3:16–17). Our bodies are temples of the Holy Spirit, and we should treat them as such. Christians tend to separate physical health in one category, mental health in another category, and spiritual health yet in another. However, I believe the scriptures teach that health in all areas is important. What is your life's purpose? What is the call of God on your life? Can you do it to its full potential if you are in poor health?

- "For one has faith to eat all things, but he who is weak eats only vegetables. Do not let him who eats despise him who does not eat, and do not let him who does not eat judge him who eats, for God has welcomed him" (Rom. 14:2–3). This topic continues for the entirety of Romans 14, but the gist is you shouldn't pass judgment on how others eat.

- "And these signs will follow those who believe: In My name they will cast out demons; they will speak with new tongues; they will take up serpents; and *if they drink anything deadly, it will by no means hurt them*; they will lay hands on the sick, and they will recover" (Mark 16:17–18, NKJV, emphasis added). This verse could be used to say we just shouldn't be concerned with what we eat or drink because in Christ we are protected. I believe in the supernatural protection of God. However, I don't think this verse gives us permission to eat or drink poorly.

When I prepare foods, raw or cooked, I use ingredients as organic and natural as possible. Some produce is organically grown without organic labeling, so it's good to know the farm your produce is grown on. Personally I do the best I can and try to maintain flexibility when eating out and traveling, but it helps tremendously to bring food along.

Whenever possible avoid genetically engineered (GE) foods comprised of genetically modified organisms (GMOs). GMO crops are staples in the Western diet; such crops include corn, sugar beets, and soy. The list continues to grow. Often mistaken for the natural selection process of hybridization, GMO crops have been genetically altered at the molecular level. Specifically, GMO crops have been genetically altered to resist glyphosate, the active ingredient commonly used by both farmers and gardeners as an herbicide. Studies show that glyphosate chelates minerals from plants and soil, immobilizing key minerals and inhibiting the key enzyme cytochrome P450 (CYP), which works to detoxify xenobiotics. Glyphosate's role as a chelator of micronutrients and ability to destroy the immune system in plants is linked to diseases and conditions in the Western diet, including diabetes, heart disease, depression, autism, infertility, birth defects, gluten intolerance, cancers, miscarriages, and obesity.[1]

Gluten is almost eliminated from my diet with the exception of the occasional bread from organic sprouted grains. Personally my digestion is better without dairy, but I find that I'm fine with fermented types of raw, organic dairy, such as kefir and yogurt. (For more on raw, unpasteurized yogurt, see chapter 5.).

I find the idea of a "do not eat list" long, restrictive, and no fun. Instead, I enjoy turning vibrant and living fruits, vegetables, nuts, and seeds into delicious juices, smoothies, salads, sides, entrées, and desserts. The diets of my students and clients have ranged the gamut of food choices. My personal approach is not to tell a person what they can or cannot eat, but rather to introduce healthy, plant-based foods that taste amazing. Whether you are raw vegan, fruitarian, Paleo, gluten-free, or just trying to eat the best you can, I hope to offer cleansing ways to reboot your system to start you on your own journey to health and wholeness.

BE DELICIOUSLY HEALTHY

After my culinary studies I returned to China ready to teach classes. With a wide repertoire of raw food recipes under my belt, I quickly discovered many of the ingredients I needed weren't available in China. The Greek philosopher Plato said,

"Necessity...is the mother of our invention" and I found that to be true.[2] I leaned on Beijing's organic farms and outdoor wet markets for a vast array of spices and exotic fruits I would use to develop recipes for classes at the local health store.

The Chinese viewed my raw vegan cuisine as a non-traditional novelty. While Chinese people eat a diet high in vegetables, they are traditionally cooked. In China, especially in the big cities of Beijing and Shanghai, a Western, fast-food diet is being adopted. It's not uncommon to see overweight Chinese, suffering from the disease of affluence, in the cities; this isn't the case when one travels into more rural areas where a traditional Chinese diet is the norm.

While most of my students and clients were European and North American expatriates, being the only raw food chef at the time in China opened up doors for me to speak at international schools and companies. Doors opened up for interviews on television on networks including Blue Ocean Network (BON TV), International Shanghai Channel (ISC), and China Central Television (CCTV), where I made raw, no-rice sushi and a chocolate layered cherry cream tart with a walnut crust. When CCTV called back for a second interview, they said they heard I made raw vegan Chinese mooncakes. I replied, "Yes, I can. When do I show up?" While the truth was I *could* make a raw version of Chinese mooncakes, in fact, I never had made them. For the next forty-eight hours I was experimenting. My roommate and official taste tester approved, and I was out the door and on my way.

UNDER THREAT

I returned to the states where I finished my first recipe book. With organic co-ops, natural food stores, and juice bars more available to the American consumer, why are people becoming more obese, disease-prone, exhausted, and sick? Are we the generation that will not outlive our parents? In addition, to meet special dietary needs of the health conscious, I started a healthy food line called Jenny's Pure Food. Gaining health does not mean giving up taste.

I've started with gluten-free, dairy-free, and low glycemic desserts: Chocolate Mousse, Lemon Cream Custard, and Salted Karmel Cheezecake. With regard to food intolerances and personal food preferences, Jenny's Pure Food gives people options. I also started classes in the Boise area, teaching raw food classes at the Boise Co-op.

News Flash

This is not a test. Repeat. This is not a test. We are under invasion by UFOs—Unidentified Frankenfood Objects. Sightings of cute, disk-shaped objects, cleverly disguised as *cookies*, *chips*, or *wafers* are being reported. They often contain genetically altered corn, soy, or sugar beets. These ETs (extra toxins) hide themselves in boxes and packages labeled "healthy," "low fat," or "low in calories." Down this rabbit hole are hidden bleached flours, refined sugars, and chemical preservatives. Read your labels. Better yet, eat foods without labels. You have been warned.

YOU MIGHT BE A FOODIE

The thought of detoxing and changing one's diet can be a frightening thing. Change can be difficult for anyone, but even more so for foodies. Foodies are those who find so much pleasure in food that life would lose its luster if their favorite restaurants, meals, and comfort foods were taken away.

Chances are you might be a foodie if:

- You read cookbooks as novels.

- You watch the *Food Network*.

- You enjoy garnishing or plating your meals.

- You enjoy strolling down each grocery aisle.

- You take pictures and post your meals for your friends to see.

However, with the recipes in this book, my aim is to make any lifestyle change in regards to food as painless as possible. As your body begins to cleanse, it will start thanking you for all the nourishment you are feeding it. This change will result in your body starting to crave different types of foods, often those rich in micronutrients, enzymes, and healing properties, such as those I introduce in this book.

A CHEF'S DILEMMA

Food is one of life's greatest pleasures, and too often the gastronomic bliss we feel from the comfort foods we love is short-lived until indigestion, heartburn, and bloating force us to ask, "Why did I eat that?" Taste, texture, and appearance are necessary components that embody good cuisine. However, what about the health aspect? Life-giving food seems to be the missing ingredient in most recipes today.

THE ROAD LESS TRAVELED

Beware of the potential pitfalls along the path to healthy eating and vibrant living. Roadblocks may come in the form of discouragement from others hindering you from making the lifestyle change to eat raw. They simply may not understand the health benefits of a raw diet, or they may fear the idea of eating fast food by themselves. Then there are those excuses: Working long hours? *Grab some junk food.* Someone criticize you at work? *You deserve a chocolate chip cookie.* Got a promotion? *Treat yourself to the dessert menu.* Hey, we've all been there. People often say we must splurge once in a while, and everything must be done in moderation. This advice sounds good because there is an element of truth in it, but don't be fooled by this group speak.

Finding balance in life is good, but the reality is people utter justifications for eating poorly because they simply have no better options available. Personally I find it hard to limit myself to just *one* refined cookie or a *single* fried chip. How about a delicious balance of fruits, vegetables, nuts, and seeds, eaten as whole foods or in mouthwatering recipes? Imagine satiating the palate with delicious foods that nourish the body.

BEAT THE SYSTEM

Choice is powerful. It is a word of responsibility. Too often it's easier to blame people or circumstances for our poor food choices. You went to that birthday party and didn't want to be rude, so you ate two hotdogs. Someone else got promoted at work, so now you deserve to eat anything you want. In short, there will always be an excuse to eat poorly.

Making a commitment to climb a mountain is more difficult than walking up one hill at a time. Often slow, small investments to your health will have the longest lasting benefits. Small steps in the right direction can lead to great victories. You can overcome even the most common of excuses and negative thoughts, including the following:

- "I don't have the time." The easiest and most time-saving way to eat is not to not cook at all! Just by having whole fruits and vegetables and nut and seed butters on hand, snacks and quick meals are pretty simple. Many of my recipes require washing, chopping, and blending to make smoothies, soups, and dressings—taking no more than ten minutes. Busy people can bring a blender to work, and some travel with their blenders.

- "I'm on a budget." Good health is not reserved for the rich. Eating well does not mean buying imported products and expensive kitchen equipment. Buying local fruits and vegetables is often less expensive than packaged and ready-made meals. Organic produce is typically more costly than conventional produce, but for those who see a link between food and health, spending a little more upfront on quality saves more on medical bills down the road. In short, you cannot afford to eat poorly.

- "I travel a lot." Business trips, road trips, and overseas excursions are wonderful opportunities to experience new flavors and textures. Traveling can break a normal routine; if traveling is part of your schedule, consider buying a travel-size version of the kitchen equipment you use most often—for me, it's a blender. Upon arrival, locate the nearest organic store, supermarket, or produce market. Don't be afraid to try new foods.

- "I don't have the willpower." Bad habits are hard to break. Remember that eating better is about making small steps in the right direction. You do not have to be militant about eating perfect; in fact, doing so often leads to the feeling of failure. Progress comes much easier with the discovery of flavors in natural ingredients that replace bad food cravings. Start with my recipes and begin to make a list of healthy alternatives to replace junk food cravings. For instance, having an apple or trail mix on hand helps prevent eating junk food on impulse.

- "I can't detox and be social." Food choices must not alienate one from friends and meeting new people. Going out to meet friends doesn't need to center around food. If you're detoxing, then simply go out for some tea and enjoy the good conversation. While most restaurants offer something healthy on the menu, options are often limited. I remind myself that fellowship is more important than my food selection, and I often drink a smoothie or put trail mix and an apple in my purse before going out. Try hosting healthy dinners and sharing recipes with friends. Lastly lecturing friends on their poor food choices (especially while they are eating) is a turn off. A little tact goes a long way and your most convincing argument will be your own glorious transformation.

- "I can't be like so-and-so." Role models and people we look up to for inspiration can be motivation to keep going, but there is no room to compare yourself to others or place them on a pedestal. Your journey of clean eating will be your own, unique experience. Your detoxification will start you on a new journey. Some may find the fruitarian diet to suit them, while others use a Paleo version. It's not only a personal choice, but the goal is to be the very best "you" and not an imitation of something, or someone, you think you should be.

CHAPTER 2

Cleansing and Detoxification: A Simple Approach to Good Health and Clean Food

P EOPLE IN THE health industry will often ask how I eat, mainly to see if my own food guidelines line up with their own philosophy on food and nutrition. I do not mind sharing my passion for getting a lot of fresh fruits and veggies into my meals while not adhering to a strict vegan or vegetarian lifestyle. Although I have studied nutrition and am passionate about health, I don't align myself with one particular diet, or one way of eating. Let's face it, there seems to be a new diet trend on the market every year. But really, it's not about me. It's about my clients and the people I help. In practice, the culinary art of matching food preferences to my clients' needs—whether it be a food intolerance or a medical-prescribed diet—is most important. Making it taste better can be a game changer.

Before addressing the art of clean eating for a detoxified lifestyle, *toxins* must first be defined. Toxins are foreign substances from chemicals in our air, water and food supply. My first encounter with toxins was before I even knew what the word *toxin* meant. In high school I read that toxins in some deodorants were linked to Alzheimer's. While I couldn't prove or disprove it, I decided that I didn't want to end up my own laboratory experiment, so I stopped using deodorant for the most part. Later I found out there are natural deodorants found in natural food stores. Then came a change in toothpaste as I opted for natural toothpastes without chemicals. I believe this concern for toxins was the beginning of my fascination with merging cuisine and health.

FOOD INTOLERANCES AND TOXICITY

There seems to be a steady wave of the new foods to avoid. Have these foods always been bad, or is this a new phenomenon? If we round up the most common food intolerances—from corn, soy, and sugar beets on the one hand to "bad" foods such as wheat, dairy, and meat on the other hand—there is much disagreement and explanation missing. Often the argument is "vegan or nonvegan," or "dairy or nondairy." But there needs to be more emphasis on clean dairy and clean meat. I consume both clean dairy and clean meat in small doses on occasion, while most days eating dairy and meat free. The main issue should be about chemical applications and genetic modifications.

Animal feed in the forms of grain and alfalfa are commonly GMO. The best way to avoid meat and dairy products with glyphosate residue is to buy organic, either labeled or from a farmer or rancher you know with organic practices. (Organic certification is expensive and time consuming. Often farmers have organic produce or animal products but are still in the process of getting certification. They may have the reputation of organic practices without having the certification.)

Corn, soy, and sugar beets: these are a few of the top foods to avoid. Assume they are all genetically modified crops (GMO) or genetically engineered (GE) unless labeled otherwise. GMO food crops are banned in much of Europe, but not the United States. There is a two-part system to such crops. Industrialized agriculture is producing both engineered plants and the toxic herbicides made in conjunction with them. The most common herbicide used in the United States. is glyphosate. It is a mineral chelator, binding up micronutrients so they are unavailable to nourish the plant.[1] Mineral chelation and micronutrient deficiency is linked to disease.[2]

There is a movement and market trend among consumers to buy non-GMO food products, often with non-GMO labeling, because they are bad for health.[3] The herbicide glyphosate is used as a GMO component (the seed is genetically altered to resist glyphosate), and the herbicide is also applied to some traditional, non-GMO crops as well, such as wheat and cane sugar. Hence, even though wheat and cane sugar are not GE (genetically engineered), they are commonly desiccated, or ripened, with glyphosate during the harvesting process and thus carry glyphosate residue with them.[4] Hence, extra measures should be taken to buy organic products when the non-organic options contain wheat and cane sugars.

According to the World Health Organization, there are five herbicides which were classified as "probably" or "possibly" carcinogenic to humans. Among these pesticides are: glyphosate, malathion, diazinon, tetrachlorvinphos, and parathion. The article points out that glyphosate is currently the most commonly used in agriculture. This article also quotes: "For the herbicide glyphosate, there was *limited evidence of carcinogenicity* in humans for non-Hodgkin lymphoma."[5] Dr. Don Huber, Professor Emeritus of Plant Pathology at Purdue University, pointed out that glyphosate is unique in that it is systemic, flowing through the leaves to the roots in plants as well being released into the soil where it binds up minerals.[6] Other diseases linked to the chelating effect of glyphosate include gastrointestinal disorders, obesity, diabetes, heart disease, depression, autism, infertility, cancer, and Alzheimer's disease.[7] What a lot to worry about! Now all the concern caused by all this information causes more toxins through stress. Fear not! By offering hope and solutions, a path to detox is attainable. Dr. Huber's personal method of detoxing glyphosate from the body is to take zeolite, specifically clinoptilolite, and humic acid.

We are exposed to increasing amounts of toxicity from the air, water, and food, whether it be industry waste, radiation, pollution from motor vehicles, or pesticides. It's difficult for our bodies to keep up with good housecleaning. Detoxification is the process by which our bodies cleanse and release wastes, poisons, and excess matter. The body was created to naturally remove toxins through the bowels, sweat glands, and skin. Fewer toxins in the system mean less work for the organs.[8]

When these toxins enter our system, it's called intestinal toxemia, the process of toxins entering the system and growing in the small and large intestines. Simply put, the bad stuff enters our gut and starts growing. Toxicity often causes symptoms of fatigue, congestion, headaches, and indigestion. While we cannot control every toxic element in our environment, we are responsible for the foods we consume, which are often bleached and refined flours, sugars, and other chemical additives. These toxins build up and manifest in the symptoms of weight gain, inflammation, and bloating, and eventually transition to more serious health problems down the road. In addition overeating and eating late at night contribute to intestinal toxemia. Hence, even if foods are healthy choices, unhealthy habits can lead to a toxic environment from a stressful lifestyle or unresolved emotional issues.[9] Many turn to dieting as a solution.

The words *diet* and *detox* are often used interchangeably. However, while the first is a quick fix weight-loss solution, cautioning us to carefully count fat grams and calories, the latter involves wholesome nutrients that cleanse and nourish the body. Weight loss, or weight gain for those who need it, can be a natural and permanent result of a healthy lifestyle. While detox programs vary in type and length, a detoxified lifestyle is one of real foods satisfying, cleansing, and nourishing from the inside out. If you are in this for the long haul, trash the crash diets, and don't toss those nutrient-dense almonds or that good-for-you, fatty avocado just yet. Detoxification can lead to a detoxified lifestyle with benefits including a better mood, clearer skin, stronger resistance to disease, mental clarity, higher energy, spiritual clarity, healthy weight, and longevity.

Non-GMO and Organic

If a food label says non-GMO, it does not imply the food is organic. If the label reads organic, then it does imply it is non-GMO. Hence, non-organic cane sugar was probably sprayed for ripening with glyphosate in the harvesting process. It is only marketed as a healthier version of sugar over beet sugar because beet sugar is GE and has chemicals applied to it.

LET'S GET THINGS MOVING

Believe me, I hoped to avoid the topic of bowel movements and colon health. After all, this is a recipe book. Nevertheless, when detox is involved, maintaining healthy bowels requires our full attention. Detoxing through the skin via acne, rashes, and other outbreaks is not the most efficient way the body cleanses— it's certainly not the most attractive either. These outward imperfections are signs the digestive tract is keeping up with incoming toxins, which is one reason healthy teenage bodies are able to detox through acne. However, whether a youth or an adult, the best way to rid the body of toxins is not through the skin, but through the bowels.

Few people discuss elimination more than people eating a diet high in raw foods. If you've been constipated for years and suddenly experience superior digestion, well, it's hard to keep quiet about it. Fresh fruits and vegetables provide abundant sources of fiber and living water (water that is from fresh fruits and vegetables and has enzymes, as opposed to still water or drinking water), working together to cleanse, purify, and nourish the digestive tract. A clogged and overburdened colon is no laughing matter and is often a sore subject. Constipation is also a sign of health problems to come and acceleration in aging. A healthy colon produces good bacteria and microorganisms called flora, but these are becoming depleted with antibiotics administered for medical purposes or in our food supply. (Introducing good bacteria back into the digestive tract will be discussed more in chapter 5.)

What is a healthy bowel movement, anyway? Is it once per day as we're often told? For those on the standard American diet (SAD), eating three meals a day may produce one sad movement. No wonder it's normal for Americans to gain an average of a pound or more a year. Less is going out than coming in. The number of healthy meals you eat should produce the same number of bowel movements, and during detoxification the number of eliminations increases all the more. When was the last time you felt your best? Was it in high school or college? Imagine your life feeling that youthful again. The good news for those suffering from constipation is that increasing the amount of raw food and fresh juices in the diet can improve digestion, control weight gain, boost overall health, and enhance beauty.

DETOX FOR BEAUTY

Start talking about achieving beautiful kidneys, a gorgeous liver, or an attractive colon through detoxification and living foods and you may get deadpan stares or rolled eyes. Don't be discouraged. There are many who earnestly care about their health and take great strides to improve their eating habits. However, for those needing more incentive, share your natural beauty secrets for silky hair and luminous skin through the detoxing powers of raw foods, and a crowd of attentive listeners may soon gather.

Raw foods beautify, detox, and nourish the outside because they are the best foods for the inside. Applying natural ingredients, such as an almond scrub to exfoliate your face or cucumbers to reduce puffy eyes, seems like a perfectly normal thing to do. Is it strange to think eating raw almonds or fresh cucumbers will have a similar effect? In contrast, applying a barbecued pork chop as a facial mask is unimaginable and would most likely produce clogged pores and breakouts. Why expect a different result by placing it between two pieces of bread and eating it?

I once moved into an apartment with kitchen walls coated in cooked oils. It took hours of scrubbing the compacted, rancid oils before a glossy white appeared. Just as these cooked oils stuck to the stovetop and frying pans, and were not easily removed with running water or a gentle wipe, so these toxins build up on the inside, clogging arteries, increasing blood pressure, and causing weight gain. If that's not bad news enough, these toxins also speed up the aging process and produce wrinkles.

In contrast to oils that undergo extreme temperatures of heat, natural oils and fats found in raw foods, on the other hand, nourish the skin and promote beauty as well as build internal health. Some of my favorite natural fats are found in avocados, coconuts, and cashews. Raw foods also help maintain healthy skin through good hydration. I hydrate best with living water from fresh fruits and vegetables—juiced, blended, or eaten whole. Most mornings I start the day off with either fruit and vegetable juice, a green smoothie, or coconut water.

IS DETOXIFICATION THE ANSWER TO OBESITY?

In America over one-third of adults and 17 percent of children are obese.[10] Throughout my travels in Europe, the Middle East, North Africa, and Asia it was much less often that I saw overweight individuals than in America, and even rarer were sightings of obesity. From 1998 to 1999, I lived in Chengdu, the capital of Sichuan Province in China's southwest region, studying at Sichuan University and interning for the US Commercial Service in Chengdu. Among the many Chinese I saw, I only remember seeing one overweight Chinese person. He happened to be Chinese American. Ten years later I was living in more modern cities, such as Beijing and Shanghai, and it was apparent that American exports were making great strides in the Chinese marketplace in the form of the fast food chains and junk food brands. While far behind the obesity problem of the United States, China is suffering from a disease of their own—the disease of affluence. With China's growing middle class, there is more expendable income to spend at convenience stores and fast food outlets located on every corner.

Weight problems can often lead to medical complications,

ranging from heart disease to gallstones to degenerative arthritis to adult-onset diabetes to cancers. The health risks of being grossly overweight can lead to drugs and surgical procedures to prevent premature death.[11] Obesity is often seen as an indication of over-nourishment counteracted by rigorous counting of calories and fat grams paralleled alongside portion control. In contrast, obesity is an epidemic of malnourishment as common food choices in diets involve artificial beverages and meals void of nutrients. Hunger pangs soon set in, and the individual succumbs to food or alcohol cravings. These repeated experiences serve as false confirmations and reminders that the individual suffers from a lack of self-will and discipline. This vicious cycle turns into the infamous yo-yo dieting.[12]

This calls into mind the famous definition from Albert Einstein, who said insanity is "doing the same thing over and over again and expecting different results."[13]

Obesity is not a sign of laziness or a lack of discipline. Genetics are certainly a part of the obesity equation. However, genetics don't help explain why obese people often have overweight pets, so lifestyle choices also come into play. According to Dr. Joel Fuhrman, a combination of food choices and physical movement along with genetics determines one's weight.[14]

It is often said we are what we eat; however, it's more what our bodies absorbed in terms of nutrients versus toxins that make up our internal health. Some dieters are on very strict food regimens but don't see results because the body is unable to take in nutrients. When toxins from the environment or pesticides and chemicals in the foods we eat enter the system and cannot get eliminated, they store up in muscle, and especially in fatty tissues, areas such as the waist, brain, breasts, and prostate gland.[15] What is needed is a reboot, or a detoxification effort, to remove blockages.

Many approach the raw-food diet as a weight-loss solution. While raw foods are certainly part of the equation in maintaining a healthy weight, eating raw foods is much more of a lifestyle choice than a short-term diet, in contrast to crash diets. Choosing to eat all raw foods for a short length of time in order to get on a healthier path or eliminate unhealthy food cravings is discussed under Practical Detox Approaches and Detoxification Through Elimination and Replacement, below. Some go a step further by doing at-home enemas or hydro colonic, types of irrigation therapies. What's needed in a detox is likened to turning on the garbage disposal to move a dirty sink's waste and accumulated matter along. Clearing out our own pipes is the first step to well-functioning organs and a digestive tract that can absorb vital nutrients.[16]

WHAT'S ALL THE TOOTIN' ABOUT GLUTEN?

With gluten-free products and ingredients storming supermarket shelves, what seemed to be a trend in the eyes of many resembles more an epidemic in grains containing gluten, such as wheat, barley, and rye. While several grains contain gluten, wheat is the ingredient found in many of today's staples from breads to crackers to traditional baked favorites. Isn't bread what many of our ancestors survived and thrived on? Even Jesus referred to himself as "the bread of life" (John 6:35). How then can something as wholesome as bread be bad? Sadly the wheat eaten in biblical times, such as Einkorn and Emmer wheat varieties, is not the wheat eaten today.[17]

William Davis's book *Wheat Belly: Lose the Wheat, Lose the Weight* explains the historical evolvement of wheat from its ancient days growing in the Middle East and being harvested in the wild to its cultivation and, later, its hybridization practices.[18] For many, going off gluten grains altogether is the best solution because both gluten intolerance and celiac disease, a more severe form of gluten intolerance where autoantibodies are the result of an immune response to undigested fragments of gluten proteins, are on the rise.[19] There's a lot of confusion about the gluten phenomenon.

The claim that grains are intrinsically bad for our health exists.[20] While much attention has been focused on the grains themselves as bad, there has been less attention on the toxic environment around them. Anthony Samsel and Stephanie Seneff propose that glyphosate, the most commonly used herbicide, is the most vital factor in both the celiac disease and gluten intolerant phenomena. Celiac disease is related to the destruction of health gut flora in the forms of lactobacilli and bifidobacteria as well as the cytochrome P450 enzymes. These are all needed in the breakdown of gluten proteins and are specifically destroyed by glyphosate residue in our food supply.[21]

When I stopped eating traditional breads, my inflammation and overall health improved, including the breakouts on my forehead. Those tissue scars on my forehead also faded with the beauty and detoxification practice of dry skin brushing. However, a few times per year I will enjoy bread from organic sprouted grains, such as Ezekiel bread, with no sign of upset, inflammation, or breakouts. This can also be attributed to eating a lot of fermented vegetables, which restores my healthy gut flora so it can break down these wheat sprouts. Whether one chooses to totally eliminate gluten, highly limit it, or find ancient grain sources is a personal choice. My pantry at home consists mainly of gluten-free grains and seeds, such as buckwheat, chia, flax, quinoa, and rice.

While the hybridization and over-refinement of gluten-containing grains, such as wheat, make it more difficult for our bodies to digest them, especially in the large amounts we eat them today, there is another factor.

Due to the chemicals and toxins in our air, water, and food supply, our digestive systems are under attack. These toxins come in multiple forms from prescribed antibiotics to over-the-counter drugs to stress, and then the attack on the digestive tract can lead to leaky gut, where undigested food, including gluten proteins, enters the bloodstream and attacks the immune system.[22]

Dr. Huber pinpoints the most commonly used chemical on plants by both farmers and gardeners with the active ingredient being glyphosate. As previously mentioned, glyphosate is banned in many European countries and labeling is mandated in sixty-four countries. But in the United States it is the chemical used in conjunction with GE crops (corn, soybeans, sugar beets, alfalfa, cotton), which are referred to as GMOs. It is also used on non-GMO crops, such as wheat, lentils, chickpeas, and cane sugar as a "ripening" agent in the harvesting process, and thus, products from these crops have relatively high glyphosate residues.[23]

As a mineral chelator, glyphosate binds to minerals from both the plant and soil it is applied to, especially iron, cobalt, molybdenum, and copper. These are the same minerals associated with the mineral deficiencies in celiac disease. Second, glyphosate kills good gut bacteria, specifically targeting lactobacilli and bifidobacteria, which are key bacteria in the breaking down of gluten proteins.[24]

According to the International Agency for Research on Cancer of the World Health Organization, insecticides and herbicides—with glyphosate being the most common—show evidence of carcinogenicity linked to glyphosate in experimental animals. "The agricultural use of glyphosate has increased sharply since the development of crops that have been genetically modified to make them resistant to glyphosate.... The general population is exposed primarily through residence near sprayed areas, home use, and diet."[25]

You should be able to tell a difference by eliminating gluten for one month; some recommend avoiding all glutinous grains for at least two months.[26] Avoiding gluten will therefore eliminate the toxins often associated with gluten.

On Food Intolerances

Many food intolerances are either related to GMO foods or glyphosate foods originally made for GMO foods, and now applied to non-GMO foods. Do not think it is a mere coincidence that the top food intolerances—

wheat, corn, soy, sugar and dairy—are affected by either GMO or glyphosate that is applied to GMO foods and some non-GMO foods as well. For example, beet sugar is GMO and therefore is treated with glyphosate made for GMO products. However, cane sugar and wheat, which are currently not GMO, are still treated with glyphosate in harvesting as a ripening agent.

DETOXIFICATION SYMPTOMS AND RESULTS

When I first started eating a high amount of raw foods, I experienced a surge of energy, lightness, and well-being. At the same time my body experienced deep cleaning as it removed years of accumulated toxins. Through this detoxification and chelation of heavy metals and toxic matter in both fat and muscle tissue, I experienced skin breakouts and fatigue (after the initial surge of energy I experienced). Noticeable to me was muscle loss in my legs. Good thing I read about detoxification before this experience. I built muscle back through gym workouts, and now when I am detoxing, I do not experience the same muscle loss. It's been a long time since I weighed myself, but I'm right around the weight I was in high school, which is ten to fifteen pounds lighter than I was in my twenties.

Healing, health, and wholeness begin to occur as the detoxification process removes obstacles. Breaking bad eating or drinking habits takes time and withdrawal symptoms—headaches, food cravings, and low energy—may last for a few days.[27] However, these symptoms can take up to six weeks for some before they start to feel better.[28] Detox symptoms and results will be different for everyone. Give yourself plenty of time for rest. If you feel lightheaded, make sure to get plenty of liquids and downtime. As toxins leave your body, you may notice a body odor or bad breath; this is just a sign that the bad stuff is leaving.[29]

PRACTICAL DETOX APPROACHES

Isn't a healthy diet good enough? Do we really need to detox? Just as the personalities of the people doing them are varied, detoxes come in different shapes and sizes. They do not, however, need to be complicated. It's simple: the longer the detox and the less fiber consumed, the deeper the cleanse. Some may do a short, one-day detox to reboot their systems, and some may do a monthlong fast of prayer and meditation on liquids, seeking clarity and direction. If you are new to fasting, I recommend trying a raw-food blend for one day or up to three days, and then see how you feel.

Progress Over Perfection

Congratulations! You are embarking on a journey to better your health as well as the health of those around you. If you fall short of your desired goals for a particular season, do not get down on yourself. Your journey to health does not have to be all-or-nothing. Small measures of change can lead to big victories. Progress is your goal and not perfection.

DETOXIFICATION THROUGH ELIMINATION AND REPLACEMENT

Eliminating certain foods or ingredients can be nearly impossible and at the very least painful when we don't know what to replace them with. If you are trying to get off gluten, for example, it's best to stay away from the baked goods aisle in grocery stores or the cookie selection in coffee shops. While the selection for those with food intolerances is getting better, the transition can be excruciating. One way is to place less emphasis on the foods one shouldn't eat and replace them with whole foods and raw fruits, vegetables, nuts, seeds, or sprouts. Eat whole or eat from the recipes in this book. In order to make eliminating a certain food sustainable, you will need to find replacements so you can survive. If you are trying to see if you are intolerant of a certain ingredient, it's best to go off of it completely for one or two months.

Here are some examples:

Omit: dairy milk

Replace with: almond, coconut, cashew, hazelnut, and hemp milks (in many cases, when unpasteurized, organic, and fermented dairies are consumed, there is not a problem; my dairy intake is limited, mostly to raw, unpasteurized milk or cream, which I'll ferment at home; see chapter 5 for more information)

Omit: animal proteins

Replace with: almonds and nuts, hemp seeds, chia seeds, quinoa, legumes

Omit: candy

Replace with: dried fruits or treats sweetened with natural sugars, such as honey, maple syrup, or coconut palm nectar (choose low glycemic candies and gums sweetened with plant-based stevia and xylitol)

Detoxification Using Raw Foods

If you are leaving the SAD, try a raw-food reboot of one, two, or three days. Remember, eating raw food is not a diet but a lifestyle of incorporating more fresh ingredients into each meal.

Phase-out plan

Have a specific goal in mind upon ending your detox. For example, for a three-day raw food program commit to making at least a small but permanent change after you have finished. For some it will be starting each morning with a green smoothie; for others will be each meal is at least 50 percent raw, etc. Because raw food is so high in vitamins, phytonutrients, and micronutrients, we are satiated faster, signaling to our body to stop eating.[30]

Want to extend your raw-food program to seven days or even a month? Go for it! People often ask how long should a detox be. The goal really is to reach a detoxed lifestyle, one of whole foods and fresh ingredients. Then there will still be times a fast is needed for spiritual and mental clarity, not to exclude the need for our organs to have a complete rest from digesting foods, even if they are clean foods.

Raw-food program

Below are some examples of potential diets while on the raw-food program. Mix and match for a one-day program, or do all three for a three-day program.

DAY ONE

Upon rising: Green Garden juice (chapter 6)
Breakfast: Green Means Go smoothie (chapter 7)
Snack: apple and almonds
Lunch: Massaged Kale salad (chapter 8)
Snack: Minty Carob Smoothie (chapter 7)
Dinner: Green Tacos With Ground Walnut (chapter 9) or salad (choose one from chapter 8)
Before bed: Ruby Red Kvass (chapter 10)

DAY TWO

Upon rising: ACV Quencher (chapter 10)
Breakfast: Kale or be Kaled (chapter 7)
Snack: celery sticks with a favorite nut butter
Lunch: salad (choose one from chapter 8) and soup (choose one from chapter 7)
Snack: trail mix (raw, unsalted almonds, cashews, goji berries)
Dinner: Holodetz with Hot Mustard (chapter 9) or just a salad (choose one from chapter 8)
Before bed: hot eucalyptus tea

DAY THREE

Upon rising: Lemon-Ginger-Goji Detox (chapter 10)

Breakfast: Red Berry Banana smoothie (chapter 7)

Snack: apple slices with favorite nut butter (there are a variety of nut and seed butters available today; however, they can also be made in a commercial blender or food processor)

Lunch: salad (choose one from chapter 8)

Snack: Carob-Hemp Protein Shake (chapter 7)

Dinner: Mac and Cheese With Beet Bacon (chapter 9) or just a salad (choose one from chapter 8)

Before bed: Rejuvenating Juice Combo (chapter 6)

Note: Drink as much water as desired.

DETOXIFICATION ON RAW-FOOD BLENDS

Our bodies and digestive tract can use a rest every now and then, even on a whole food and raw-food diet. Ever eat one too many cashew cheesecakes? Ever get stevia soda sloshed or kale chip faced? Consider doing a raw-food blended detox on a monthly basis or as often as needed. By blending our food, our digestive tract is doing less work while getting all the fiber in whole foods. Feel free to warm some of the broths and soups, especially in the colder months. To do a strictly blended detox or fast, feel free to omit the whole food garnishes from the broth and soup recipes. If you want to have a deeper cleansing experience during your raw-food blended program, choose recipes with higher amounts of fruits and vegetables and fewer nuts and seeds.

Raw-food blends program

The following are some examples of potential diets while on the raw-food blends program. Mix and match for a one-day program, or do all three for a three-day program.

DAY ONE

Upon rising: For the Love of Beet juice (chapter 6)
Breakfast: Enzyme Releaser smoothie (chapter 7)
Lunch: Creamy Broccoflower (chapter 7)
Dinner: Strawberry and Black Sesame smoothie (chapter 7)
Before bed: hot tea

DAY TWO

Upon rising: Peared With Zucchini juice (chapter 6)
Breakfast: Kiwi-Spinach Cleanser (chapter 7)
Lunch: Butternut Squash soup (chapter 7)
Dinner: 4Bs: Buckwheat, Berries, Bananas, and (Nut) Butter smoothie (chapter 7)
Before bed: hot tea

DAY THREE

Upon rising: Sweet Greens juice (chapter 6)
Breakfast: Grapefruit-Goji Detox (chapter 7)
Lunch: Curried Coconut-Mango bisque (chapter 7)
Dinner: Berry Yogurt Smoothie (chapter 7)
Before bed: hot tea

CHAPTER 3

The Fast and the Curious: The Benefits of Fasting

ETOXIFICATION AND FASTING are often used interchangeably because they commonly share similar results for improved health, rejuvenation, and regeneration. While the two can be done simultaneously, distinctions rooted in consumption, motivation, and purpose exist between them.

Detoxification involves elements of cleansing with raw foods, fresh juices, herbs, or water to remove toxins from the body. While fasting may use similar elements of sustenance, it is different in that it focuses on the abstinence of certain foods or liquids in combination with prayer and meditation for breakthrough or spiritual insight. Practiced for thousands of years for both spiritual and medicinal purposes, fasting is common in every region of the world. Jesus fasted forty days in the wilderness without food or water. (See Matthew 4:1–11.) As toxins leave the body, improved health can have mental, physical and spiritual results. Cleansing can uncover and expose toxins created by stress, unforgiveness, and even bitterness. (See Hebrews 12:12–15.)

Today fasting has taken on unique and creative forms, such as fasting from watching television, playing video games, or using social media. Historically, however, the tradition of fasting involves abstinence of food to suppress physical needs to receive spiritual insight, protection, or provision. Some Christians believe food is unrelated to spiritual health since we are no longer living under the Law. While Old Testament teachings forbade eating pork, for instance, Christians are now free to eat anything at will. "All things are lawful for me, but not all things are helpful; all things are lawful for me, but not all things edify" (1 Cor. 10:23).

Hence, although eating hot dogs and marshmallow salad at the church potluck is lawful, the question remains if it is beneficial. Don't get me wrong; I'm not promoting militant eating with strict legalistic guidelines. But is there a link between the physicality of foods and spiritual awareness? I believe the ancient Scriptures point that way.

A FASTED LIFESTYLE

Some will choose a fasted lifestyle by fasting one day per week. Others may choose to eliminate a certain food item for a month at a time. Some may skip a meal, such as dinner, so they fast daily for fifteen hours or longer, counting the later afternoon until the time they awake.[1]

This partial fasting or a fasted lifestyle may be different from person to person. Desiring to live like this, I started doing forty-day partial fasts where I stop eating at 2:00 p.m. At first this was difficult to do. I literally counted the minutes to two o'clock, stuffing my face before the dreaded time reached, and then feeling deprived after 2:00 p.m. I would sometimes wake at midnight and eat something, justifying it by saying it was the morning of the next day. As I continued to do these fasts, it got easier. Soon breakfast, lunch, and a snack were all I needed to eat. The health benefits have included tremendous improvements in digestion, mental clarity, energy levels, and sleep quality. After I completed the first forty-day partial fast and returned to eating after 2:00 p.m., I noticed a huge difference in how I felt. I felt much better while on the fast. Hence, I've tried to do several of these since with the goal of making this a lifestyle with some exceptions allowed, especially for special occasions. It was important for me not to let these times of partial fasting affect my quality time with friends and family or keep me from meeting new people. However, going to parties and dinners has often become more about the people, the conversations, and the interactions rather than just the food. I don't feel the need to do these partial fasts as a form of legalism, but in order to create a lifestyle and habit I found that having a forty-day goal written down on a calendar helps.

FASTING AND FOOD IN THE BIBLE

Complete health involves three parts: spiritual health, mental health, and physical health. Too many Christians focus solely on spiritual health to the detriment of physical and mental health. The Bible speaks of physical health and its importance as well, however.

John wrote: "Beloved, I pray that all may go well with you and that you may be in good health, even as your soul is well" (3 John 2). Verse 3 mentions that Christians "walk in truth." I urge you to not only walk in spiritual truth, but also to walk in truth in regards to your food. Knowing the truth about what you are eating, about GMOs, and about chemicals in food is necessary.

The story of Daniel goes into more detail about the foods Daniel ate, and it is a popular diet for people to follow today. In the Old Testament, Daniel, a Jewish boy taken captive into Babylon, now modern-day Iraq, was chosen among a select group of young men to be trained to serve the king. These young men were selected based on their appearance, physique, and ability to learn in wisdom, knowledge, and understanding. They would learn the language and literature of the Chaldeans (Dan. 1:4).

The first mention of Daniel fasting in the book of Daniel reads:

> The king appointed them a daily provision of the king's food and of the wine which he drank. They were to be educated for three years, that at the end of it they might serve before the king. . . . But Daniel purposed in his heart that he would not defile himself with the portion of the king's food, nor with the wine which he drank. Therefore he requested of the master of the officials that he might not defile himself. Now God had brought Daniel into favor and compassion with the master of the officials. The master of the

officials said to Daniel, "I fear my lord the king who has appointed your food and your drink. For why should he see your faces worse-looking than the youths who are your age? Then you would endanger my head before the king."

Then Daniel said to the steward, whom the master of the officials had set over Daniel, Hananiah, Mishael, and Azariah, "Please test your servants for ten days, and let them give us vegetables to eat and water to drink. Then let our countenances be looked upon before you, and the countenance of the youths who eat of the portion of the king's food. And as you see, deal with your servants." So he consented to them in this matter and tested them for ten days.

At the end of ten days their countenances appeared fairer and fatter than all the youths who ate the portion of the king's food. Thus the guard continued to take away the portion of their food and the wine that they were to drink, and gave them vegetables.

—Daniel 1:5, 8–16

Today this is often referred to as the Daniel Fast, but seldom do people take this part in context, as Daniel's fast was a ten-day trial period to prove a fasted lifestyle that lasted three years or longer, depending on how long he stuck to vegetables and water (Dan. 1:5–8). Put into today's practical application, a ten-day trial could be seen as a jumpstart into eating healthier, not as a short-term diet, but as a reboot to a better plan long-term, proving to yourself, your doctor, or someone else that the changes made in a ten-day trial period helped.

So on one side Christians interpret the Daniel Fast as a short-term eating plan. On the other side, this plant-based diet is often used to promote a vegan lifestyle. From Scripture I believe it is safe to assume Daniel went for a long period of time, perhaps months or years at a time, surviving and thriving on a plant-based diet but without adhering to a strict vegan diet. In Scripture Daniel goes on another fast, eating "no tasty food, no meat or wine" to mourn over a disturbing vision he was shown of future events to come (Dan. 10:3). Daniel abstaining from meat for a period of time implies that Daniel was not always eating a vegan diet and that he was conscientious about what he put in his body, and we can benefit from mirroring his lifestyle.

> As for these four youths, God gave them knowledge and skill in every branch of learning and wisdom. And Daniel had understanding in all kinds of visions and dreams.
>
> —DANIEL 1:17

Beyond promoting good health, the connection between fasting and seeking God and being more alert to the supernatural realms is evident in Daniel's life. What about miracles? There is a story in the New Testament when Jesus's disciples were unable to heal an epileptic suffering from a demon and, instead, Jesus rebuked the demon and healed him. When the disciples asked him why they were not able to heal the boy, He said it was because of unbelief and that prayer and fasting were key (Matt. 17:20–21).

Have you ever needed a breakthrough? Have you ever sought God in desperation for a miracle? There is another example from Scripture where Esther and her people fasted, neither eating nor drinking for three straight days, to seek God for breakthrough, favor, and protection on behalf of the Jewish nation, which was in exile and in danger of being annihilated (Esther 4:15–17).

BEGINNING AND ENDING A FAST: PHASE-IN AND PHASE-OUT STRATEGY

You just cleansed and feel great. This good feeling ends the day you return to your SAD (standard American diet). Unfortunately too many fasts do more damage than good. How can this be? Sometimes good intentions reap unhealthy rewards. For starters, fasting is no quick-fix diet plan. Drinking empty-calories pumped with caffeinated stimulants, refined sweeteners, and chemical additives on an empty system is harmful and resembles more of an eating disorder than the life-giving benefits of fasting.

In addition, many break a fast only to experience indigestion and discomfort worse than before they started. This happens because once the organs and digestive tract are clean, now accustomed to pure water, fresh juices, or raw foods, they often encounter surprise attacks by processed foods or UFOs—unidentified Frankenfood objects—due to their enlightened sensitivity to chemicals, antibiotics, and preservatives in foods. One may even discover an existing food allergy to a particular type of food just because the system is now clean enough to feel the difference.

Feel free to start a water or juice fast anytime you feel like it. However, I personally find that one to three days of blended smoothies and soups before I begin a juice fast helps me ease into drinking only juices. Likewise, to help me come out of a juice or water fast, I've found that either raw fruits or blended smoothies and soups are a gentle way of introducing whole foods back into the system. If someone is eating the normal SAD diet of processed foods and conventional dairy and meats (non-organic, not grass-fed) and wants to do a juice or water fast, it may be helpful to "ease-in" and "ease-out" of the fast by eating raw foods for one, two, or three days before and after the fast. After the fast, go from blended smoothies and soups to whole and raw foods. By now your body should be clean enough to tell you when you eat something it does like or tolerate. For some this could be wheat products; for others it could be dairy or soy.

A good way to end, or even begin, a water or juice fast is to drink blended fruits and vegetables, such as the smoothies and soups in this book. Gradually work up to eating solid foods, keeping them as natural and organic as possible. This can help curb the side effects of a higher sensitivity to chemicals, antibiotics, and preservatives.

Many succeed on detox programs and juice and smoothie fasts, experiencing results of weight loss, more energy, clearer thinking, and a better mood (not to mention clothes starting to fit again). Nevertheless, this experience is short-lived because people have no idea what to do when it's all over. This is why I provided a raw food menu of international cuisines at the end of this book. Getting plenty of clean fruits and veggies into your daily routine will help you maintain a detoxed lifestyle. Remember, it's not an all-or-nothing approach, but if you go back to your same old habits you will get the same old results!

GETTING ENOUGH REST

Rest is essential to health, and it's even more important during a fast. As the organs and digestive tract begin to deep clean, give the body plenty of time to do its job. Of course, if you are "fasting" from watching too much television or from eating meat, then your body probably will not need extra rest. However, if you are doing a juice fast it's important to slow way down. Personally I find if I do a smoothie fast for one to three days, I can carry on with a normal schedule.

In today's fast-paced world many people feel they cannot afford to take one day off per week to rest. The pressures and expectations to work around the clock, however, can catch up with a person, leading to burn out and sickness. Resting in general, in combination with detoxing and fasting, can help a person's health. I find that taking a day to rest my mind, soul, and body not only increases my productivity level throughout the week, but also improves my mood and overall outlook on life. I used to look at the morning as the beginning of my day and feel flustered at all the things I had to accomplish. Then I started to see the start of my day at sunset, the evening before. I would make a list of priorities for the following morning, and this changed my perspective and routine. Getting enough rest also curbs overeating; in contrast, a lack of sleep promotes premature aging.[2]

JUICE FASTING

During a juice fast, no fibers are consumed, just juices and their rich nutrients. This gives our organs an easier time digesting what we do consume and thus a deeper cleansing effect. I learned to make my fasts more comfortable by using the phase in and phase out method. Can you go longer than a one-day juice fast? Yes, but make sure to give yourself plenty of time to rest throughout the fast.

Fasting plan: one-day juice fast (with phase-in and phase-out)

- The day before (phase-in): eat only whole fruits or veggies *or* only fresh juices (herbal teas and broths OK)

- Fast: fresh juices (herbal teas and broths OK)

- Day after (phase-out): eat only whole fruits or veggies *or* only fresh juices (herbal teas and broths OK)

- The day after phase-out will be the day you may be hungriest and craving foods that will counteract the benefits of your juice fast. During this time I highly recommend not watching the Food Network or looking at food pictures on Pinterest or Instagram. Your mind may play tricks on you. During one detox I started craving blueberry muffins, a food I typically would not crave. When this happens, don't give in. Keep going.

Example one-day juice program (with phase-in and phase-out)
>Phase-in: day before
>Heavier phase-in: raw-food meals
>Medium phase-in: raw foods eaten whole
>Lighter phase-in: blended smoothies and soups

JUICE DAY
>Upon rising: Green Light Infusion (chapter 6)
>Breakfast: Grape Expectations (chapter 6)
>Mid-morning: Cleansing Miso Broth (chapter 7)
>Lunch: Citrus Regenerator (chapter 6)
>Afternoon: Spicy Tomato Broth (chapter 7)
>Dinner: Green Supreme (chapter 6)
>Before bedtime: tea
>Phase out: day after
>Heavier phase-out: raw-food meals
>Medium phase-out: raw foods eaten whole
>Lighter phase-out: blended smoothies and soups

Prepare your juices and blends as close to consumption as possible. Double up on these juices and broths at will! Are you too busy to juice? You can juice everything at once or the day before as you should be resting as much as possible. Another option is to order your day's worth of juices from the local co-op by calling forty-eight hours in advance to place your order. (Many areas have local co-ops. Some are listed at www.ncg.coop.) Otherwise, you can just order your daily juice at the counter without calling ahead. Add in water when you feel like it throughout your juice fasts. After you have successfully completed a one-day juice fast, try three days.

WATER FASTING

Begin with a one-day fast, but plan for three-days total, with one phase-in day and one phase-out day. During the fast, no fibers are consumed. This gives our organs an even easier time in digesting and thus a deeper cleansing effect. Make sure to phase in and phase out of water fasts; doing so can certainly make your fast more comfortable. Can you go longer than a one-day fast? Yes, but give yourself plenty of time to rest.

Fasting plan: one-day water fast (with phase-in and phase-out)

- Day before (phase-in): drink only smoothies or juices (herbal teas and broths OK)

- Fast: water only (including rejuvelac or coconut water)

- Day after (phase-out): drink only smoothies or juices (herbal teas and broths OK)

If you do a longer fast, such as a three-day juice or water fast, you can still use the one-day phase-in and phase-out plan.

CHAPTER 4

Raw Food Basics: Shopping List and Tips

THIS CHAPTER PROVIDES a shopping list and tips to get you started eating raw and healthily. The shopping list provides most of the food and kitchen tools needed for the recipes in this book. Your range of produce will vary depending on your geographical location and seasonal selection. For this reason, when I list specific types and varieties of produce—such as shiitake mushrooms, roma tomatoes, or Granny Smith apples—feel free to use the produce that's on sale at your natural foods store or in season at your local farmer's market. The transition and sustainability of your eating more living foods depend on the simplicity and ease in making the recipes as well as sourcing affordable and accessible produce. Hence, use this list as a guideline.

Produce marked with an asterisk should be stored on the countertop. When countertop produce reaches its ripeness, it's time to eat it or move it to the refrigerator to slow down the ripening process. Nuts and seeds can be refrigerated, but if the weather is cool they can be stored in the pantry. Cold-pressed oils are heat-sensitive, and storing them in the refrigerator gives them a longer shelf life. If oils smell rancid, discard them.

Coconut oil is an exception to the refrigeration rule; it can be stored in the pantry due to its stability in cool temperatures. Coconut oil is often solid; it liquefies around 75 degrees Fahrenheit. If the weather is warm, move the coconut oil to the refrigerator. When my recipes call for coconut oil, this means coconut oil in liquefied form. To liquefy, add the amount needed to a bowl and place the bowl inside a larger bowl of hot water for a few minutes.

SHOPPING LIST

Produce	
Apples	Avocados*
Bananas*	Beetroots
Blackberries	Blueberries
Broccoli	Cabbage
Carrots	Cauliflower
Celery	Cherries
Cherry tomatoes	Coconuts*
Corn (sweet)	Cucumbers
Eggplants	Garlic
Ginger	Jicama root
Lemons*	Limes*
Mangos*	Mushrooms (button, cremini, shiitake, etc.)
Onions*	Oranges*
Pears	Peppers (bell, jalapeño, habanero, etc.)
Potatoes	Radishes
Raspberries	Sprouts (alfalfa, broccoli, mung beans, soybean, etc.)
Strawberries	Tomatoes
Turmeric root	Watermelon*
Zucchini	
Leafy Greens and Herbs	
Basil	Cilantro
Collard greens	Dill

Detox Delish

Green onions	Kale
Parsley	Peppermint
Romaine lettuce	Spinach
Spices	
Allspice	Black pepper
Cayenne	Chili
Cinnamon	Curry powder
Garlic powder	Nutmeg
Onion powder	White pepper
Dried fruits, nuts, and seeds	
Almonds	Buckwheat
Cashews	Chia seeds
Coconut flour or shreds	Dates (honey, medjool)
Flax seeds	Macadamia nuts
Pecans	Pine nuts
Pistachios	Pumpkin seeds
Quinoa	Raisins
Sesame seeds (black and white)	Sun-dried tomatoes
Sunflower seeds	Walnuts
Cold-pressed oils	
Cacao butter	Coconut oil
Flaxseed oil	Olive oil
Sesame oil (toasted is OK; it is hard to find cold-pressed)	
Sweeteners	
Coconut palm nectar	Dried fruit

Maple syrup	Raw honey
Stevia	

Other	
Agar powder	Apple cider vinegar
Cacao powder	Carob powder
Chlorella powder	Goji berries
Green clay (food grade)	Kelp powder
Lecithin (soy or sunflower)	Maca powder
Matcha powder (Green tea powder)	Miso (chickpea or soy)
Natural soy sauce (gluten-free tamari or coconut soy-free aminos)	Nori seaweed sheets
Nutritional yeast	Reishi powder
Sea salt	Spirulina powder
Vanilla extract	

Herbal detox teas	
Alfalfa	Dandelion flower
Dandelion root	Eucalyptus
Goji berries	Hawthorn berries
Juniper berries	Marshmallow root
Milk thistle	Turmeric, fresh or dried

Kitchen equipment	
Blender	Food processor
Food dehydrator	Juicer
Kitchen tools	8- or 10-inch chef's knife
9-inch pie plate	9-inch spring form pan

9-inch tart pan	Bamboo sushi mat
Grater	Kitchen scissors
Lemon press or handheld juicer	Measuring cups and spoons
Melon ball scooper	Mixing bowls
Nut milk bag or cheesecloth	Paper towels
Parchment paper	Paring knife
Peeler	Rubber spatula
Serrated knife	Spiral slicer (optional)
Strainer	Toothpicks
Wooden cutting board	

ON ORGANIC

The best food to eat is organic food grown at home. The next best thing is to buy locally grown, organic produce. The first two options are not always possible, so look for foods with organic labels in stores. Keep in mind that eating organic does not have to be an all-or-nothing approach. It's especially difficult when traveling or eating at restaurants, so do the best you can.

In order to avoid buying conventional produce with the highest pesticide residues, follow this list of the "dirty dozen" plus a couple more. These are the foods that it is most important to buy organic:

1. Apples

2. Cherry tomatoes

3. Potatoes

4. Peaches

5. Celery

6. Cherries

7. Collard greens

8. Cucumbers

9. Grapes (imported)

10. Kale

11. Lettuce

12. Nectarines

13. Pears

14. Snap Peas

15. Spinach

16. Strawberries

17. Sweet bell peppers[1]

Here are the clean fifteen, the fifteen foods that have the lowest pesticide found in testing and therefore are OK to eat if you don't buy organic:

1. Asparagus

2. Avocados

3. Cabbage

4. Cantaloupe

5. Cauliflower

6. Eggplant

7. Grapefruit

8. Kiwi

9. Mangos

10. Onions

11. Papayas[2]

12. Pineapples

13. Sweet corn[3]

14. Sweet peas

15. Sweet potatoes[4]

ON WASHING PRODUCE

I typically give my produce a good rinse or scrub. You can also soak produce for ten to fifteen minutes in a tub of water with a few splashes of apple cider vinegar, which works as a natural antibacterial disinfectant, and then rinse. There are also several products to wash produce. Use brands containing chemical-free and all-natural ingredients.

ON CUTTING BOARDS

Choose wooden cutting boards over plastic. Not only are there natural properties to fight bacteria in wooden cutting boards, but also they do not dull knives like plastic cutting boards do. Any type of cross-contamination must be avoided. Since the recipes in this book call for fruits, vegetables, nuts, and seeds, there should be no cross-contamination with animal products. If your wooden board is not treated (does not have a glossy finish), moisturize it with coconut oil as needed.

ON SWEETENERS

Sweeteners used in my recipes include dried fruits, raw honey, maple syrup, and coconut palm nectar. Some recipes will simply call for a "liquid sweetener" due to personal preferences, from vegans (no honey) to people watching their sugar levels. When I call for a liquid sweetener, use whichever you prefer from my list. The exception to the amount used of a liquid sweetener is stevia, which is administered in drop size amounts because it is much stronger. Typically, you should use two drops stevia to one tablespoon of a liquid sweetener. However, stevia is so strong that it is better to put in a couple drops at a time and do a taste test.

Raw honey is unrefined and unprocessed. It's known for its antibacterial, antiviral, and enzymatic properties. Depending on your dietary needs and personal preferences, honey can be interchanged with other natural sweeteners.

Maple syrup is an amber-colored liquid derived from the sap of maple trees that carries a deep, woody flavor. Maple syrup, and sometimes agave nectar, is not considered raw because heat is used in the extraction process.

Coconut nectar is produced from the sap of the coconut palm, traditionally used in southern Asia and Southeast Asia. It is known for its low glycemic properties, which is better for those on a low-sugar diet.

For those watching their sugar intake, feel free to replace each tablespoon of liquid sweetener with three to five drops of liquid stevia for recipes in the smoothie and raw-ktail sections. Taste test every two drops.

ON SALT

Studies indicate that Americans consume five to ten times the sodium they need, contributing to high blood pressure and heart disease. According to Dr. Fuhrman, salt should be eliminated from the diet for optimal health.[5] Author David Wolfe defines consuming sea salt or rock salt as an anabolic (literally "to build up") process slowing down detoxification.[6]

Growing up, I actually thought meat was naturally salty. The fact is, meats are loaded with salt and sodium nitrites, which give deli meats a pink coloration. Using unbleached, mineral sea salts is a better option in foods, especially as one transitions from a high salt diet. If you are wondering whether you're consuming too much salt, if you are eating out or buying processed and pre-packaged foods you are most likely a prime candidate for cutting it down.

We have heard how vital salt is in the diet, but it's important to state that table salt is sodium chloride. Cutting out salt does not mean forgoing organic sodium sources found in foods, such as sea vegetables, celery, and spinach. Avoid table salt for a few days and you will be amazed how your senses detect the saltiness in a piece of celery.[7]

High amounts of table salt make me feel and look swollen. While I'll do almost anything for my health, I'm even more willing when it comes to beauty. Hence, I'm on a journey to use less and less table salt. I still use minimal amounts of sea salt in recipes, and many of the healthier raw and vegan snacks I enjoy also contain sea salt. I also use it to aid in the preservation of fermented vegetables. Salt is not vital in the fermentation process, but it has been traditionally used in generations past. If you are detoxing from a SAD, transitioning from the bleached salt in most processed foods to using some pink or grey-toned sea salts is an option. Still, for all the recipes in this book, sea salt will remain optional and a personal choice. You can use kelp powder in place of sea salt in recipes by experiment to see if you like the taste. In savory dishes, soups, and salads, I love the taste of seaweeds.

On Water

Chemicals in the air, used on our farmland, or dumped in landfills end up in our water systems. Rain can wash toxic chemicals into our water systems, and the chemicals end up in our drinking water. Chlorine is added to destroy microorganisms. Chlorine kills many bacteria, but it does not kill viruses and parasites.[8]

Drinking pure water helps detox and maintain healthy organs and skin. Good hydration is vital to our systems and helps keep our skin nice, plump, and supple rather than sagging and wilted. Wolfe talks about the importance of pure water, the best being living water from deep springs as part of detoxification and everyday hydration.[9] However, just what type of water is best to drink and, equally important, to detox with is up for debate.

Most of us don't walk outside each morning and fill up our jugs of natural spring water. However, we do have choices.

When I lived overseas, finding good water was a challenge. In one of the places I have lived, I've been told the five-gallon containers of water have just been refilled with tap water and resold. Later, I learned how to make rejuvelac, a probiotic beverage made from sprouted grains or seeds. Rejuvelac is a living and active water that not only offers beneficial enzymes, minerals, and probiotics, but the sprouted grains and seeds also work to filter out impurities and toxins in the water. Unfortunately pure water is a challenge in developed areas, including here at home.[10]

Today I start with pure water and use the rejuvelac process as a second filtration system to clean the water, and then discard the sprouted grains after the third batch of water. When I returned home, I reverted to filtering tap water by making rejuvelac. However, due to contamination in our water systems of arsenic, insoluble calcium, nitrates, lead, and even toilet paper residues, I was compelled to switch back to buying pure water from the local co-op down the street and then either drinking that or starting from pure water to make rejuvelac.

Now that I live so close to an organic co-op, I've gotten spoiled with choice. They have deionized water, which is so pure it's nothing but water. It's similar in purity to distilled water, and ideal for fasts and special diets. They also have reverse osmosis water, which is a drinking water with just trace amounts of minerals, devoid of chlorine and 98 percent of contaminates. Author Tonya Zavasta teaches in her book *Quantum Eating* that the best hydration is water from living foods. Keep in mind that it is virtually impossible to go without still water for most people. Fruitarians and complete raw foodists may be able to consume only living water, but most people are unable to. The water you choose is up to you. For optimal digestion it is best to drink water thirty minutes before eating and then wait one hour after eating until drinking again. If it's too hard to do this, it's because it's

Detox Delish

simply habit to drink a beverage at a meal or the food is way too
salty.

This is one reason I often have the choice of using water,
coconut water, or rejuvelac in my drinks and blended recipes.
Personally, my goal is to drink less and less still water, and
consume the majority of my water from fresh juices, coconut
water, fruits, vegetables, and rejuvelac. But for now, I still drink
deionized water from the local co-op.

GLOSSARY OF INGREDIENTS

Agar powder—Agar is derived from seaweed (red marine algae) and
   used as a vegetable gelatin to thicken foods, such as puddings
   and desserts. Agar comes in flake and stick form. In the recipes
   in this book the powder form will be used as it takes the least
   amount of time to form the gel when mixed with water.

Apple cider vinegar—Adding a zing to many salads, dressings, and
   sauces, apple cider vinegar is known for its healing properties,
   enzymes, friendly-bacteria, and amino acids. Many use it to aid
   digestion and treat diabetes and weight issues. Look for brands
   that are organic, unfiltered, unheated, and unpasteurized.

Bentonite clay—This is an absorbent clay known for powerful detox
   and chelating of toxins and heavy metals.

Cacao butter—Cacao butter is the natural oil extracted from the cacao
   bean. It has a rich white-chocolate flavor. It is often sold in solid
   blocks or in solid pieces and looks similar to beeswax. It can be
   stored in a cool, dry place or the refrigerator.

Cacao powder—Derived from the cacao bean, cacao powder is chocolate in its purest form. Cacao powder comes in toasted and raw
   forms. Raw cacao is hailed as a superfood for its rich mineral
   content and abundance of antioxidants. However, cacao can act
   as a stimulant, and some use it sparingly or substitute it with
   carob powder.

Carob powder—A mineral-rich substance from the carob pod, which
   is derived from the carob tree, carob is sweeter and less bitter
   than cacao. Although carob has a distinctly different flavor than
   cacao, they are often used interchangeably in recipes. Carob
   powder also comes in toasted and raw forms.

Chlorella powder—A green algae known for its nutrient density, chlorella is rich in vitamins, minerals, amino acids (proteins), and chlorophyll. It also aids in ridding the body of toxins and heavy metals.

Liquid aminos—This is a natural and fermented soy sauce from organic soybeans (or a soy-free sauce derived from coconuts). This gluten-free, liquid protein concentrate is great in soups, dressings, and dips. Look for organic and non-organic GMO-free brands.

Maca powder—A Peruvian root known for enhancing stamina and energy, maca powder adds a wonderful malty flavor and creaminess to milkshakes and desserts. Traditionally it was used to increase fertility in women and boost libido in men.

Miso—This is traditionally a fermented soybean paste used in many Asian cuisines for its depth of flavor and saltiness. However, your organic market may also have a non-soy variety made from chickpeas. A favorite type of miso is Japanese light-colored miso. Look for organic and non-GMO brands.

Nutritional yeast—Coming in powder or flakes, nutritional yeast is commonly mistaken for brewer's yeast. Despite its unappealing name, nutritional yeast boasts a nutty, cheesy flavor. It is known for its amino acids (proteins) and B-complex vitamins.

Psyllium husk—This is a good, water-soluble source of fiber that is often an ingredient in colon cleanses.

Seaweeds—These are a rich source of iodine and other trace minerals. Dulse, kelp, nori, and wakame are all different types of seaweeds. Their natural sodium content makes them a good alternative for adding a savory touch. Feel free to use kelp powder in place of sea salt in the recipes. You'll have to experiment to see if you like the taste in savory dishes, soups, and salads. I love the taste of seaweeds.

Tamari—A natural soy sauce, this gluten-free, liquid protein concentrate is great in soups, dressings, and dips. Look for organic and non-GMO brands. It is often used in place of traditional soy sauce or liquid aminos.

CHAPTER 5

Fermentation and Probiotics: It's Alive!

*I*F THE THOUGHT of bacteria scares you, the opposite, no bacteria, should be even more frightening. A healthy gut is abundant with intestinal flora. We are constantly surrounded by both good and bad bacteria. What is important to know about the power of cultured vegetables is that the acidifying bacteria (good stuff) multiplies quickly and is able to destroy and stop the proliferation of pathogenic organisms (bad stuff) that get in its way. Isn't it cool that when the world—including our bodies— is in balance, the good always conquers the bad? With today's modern diet and the amount of antibiotics taken, our defense system is threatened and depleted.

Before refrigeration, the development of canning, and chemical additives, societies around the world didn't just know the basics in preserving food—they were masters at their craft, preserving live food cultures through fermentation and curing. From the power of *pao cai* (Chinese) to the sensation of *sauerkraut* (German) to the keenness of *kimchee* (Korean), people around the world have perfected their living cultured delicacies in numerous forms: miso, yogurt, kefir, and cultured vegetables. To say there are hundreds of fermentation methods is an understatement.

Preparing fermented foods involves the process of breaking down substances through a heatless form of cooking, keeping the food in a raw state. Historically, these fermented live cultures offered sustenance through cold winter months when less vegetation was available. Fermentation extends beyond plant foods, however, to meat and dairy products.

Mention the importance of good bacteria and probiotics in a

diet and nine times out of ten people will mention how they eat yogurt. Ironically most yogurts come in non-organic, pasteurized form. The animals are being fed GMOs, not to mention given antibiotics and hormones. This is a major reason why our guts are so depleted of good flora today. This doesn't mean eating yogurt is bad, but conventional yogurt is inferior to how fermented dairy products have been made throughout history.

This section will focus on the basics of fermented vegetables, brines, and milks. (Check out chapter 9 for the recipes for Low-Salt Kimchee and Pickled Raw Beets.) Not only is fermentation useful for preservation purposes, but the process of making live cultures also promotes healing properties and nutrient availability. For instance, fermented vegetables, such as sauerkraut, are a rich source of vitamin C because fermentation slows down its degeneration process.[1]

In addition, the nutrients in live food cultures are also more bioavailable because the fats, proteins, and carbohydrates are broken down and pre-digested before consumption. This means less work for your digestive tract because the enzymes are working and the nutrients are more easily absorbed. Once ingested, these lactic acid foods make the bowels slightly acidic, which is needed for a healthy colon.[2] Élie Metchnikoff, a famous Russian scientist, attributed high lactic acid foods to longevity through his studies of well-aged Russians. Ferments are also said to prevent and treat diseases, including cancers and candida.[3]

Overall, fermented foods are superfoods when it comes to people dealing with gut issues. Additional benefits include decreased inflammation, improved digestion, and a strengthened immune system. This is all part of the detoxification process. There is evidence that fermented foods chelate heavy metals, such as mercury, from the body.[4]

Probiotic strains can be purchased in supplement form in health food stores. Nevertheless, there is no comparison in terms of quality, as well as quantity, of probiotics and microbes eaten directly from cultured foods—not to mention savings to your pocketbook. Unfortunately many ferments sold on the shelf are packaged and pasteurized, so your best option is to make them at home.[5] You may be surprised at how easy a simple cabbage kraut is to make and how eating small portions at a time can go a long way. I once made a red cabbage kraut that lasted a year in pristine condition. Fermented foods bring an array of edginess, sharpness, and savory factors to many of my meals just by adding a couple spoonfuls to rice, salads, and soups.

BASIC STEPS IN FERMENTING VEGETABLES

In addition to the fermented vegetable recipes provided in this book, here are steps to help you get started in your fermenting adventures:

Select your produce

Cabbage is one of the most popular vegetables to ferment. Try carrots, beets, radishes, onions, peppers, or even watermelon rinds. There is no limit to your choices, but I tend to use produce with a high water content so they can ferment in their own juices. If I use leafy greens and herbs, I'll add these to my kraut in smaller amounts for an accent of color, flavor, and nutrients.

Prep your vegetable

After washing, and scrubbing if needed, chop your vegetables into the desired size. Some krauts are not chopped at all, but maintain the vegetable in its whole form. My favorite fermented vegetables are often finely sliced, such as shredded cabbage or grated carrots, beets, and radishes.

Salt your vegetables

There are two main methods to salt your vegetables: the dry-salt method and the brine method. While adding salt helps in the preservation and fermentation process, salt is not absolutely needed. You can either omit the salt or use it in very low amounts. This is what I do since I'm trying to get much of my sodium through whole foods, such as sodium-rich celery, coconut water, and sea vegetables. When I do use salt, I use sea salt, a natural salt often colored with pink and grey tones. Sea salt is not to be mistaken for common table salt, which is stripped of trace minerals through a chemical bleaching process. Adding even modest amounts of salt does, however, enhance the taste and is believed to help the ferment last longer.[6]

Dry-salt method

After prepping your vegetables, place salt directly on the vegetables. It's a good idea to underestimate the salt amount. If a recipe calls for a certain amount of salt it's best to start with half the amount as every bunch of this and every head of that varies in size, weight, and amount. Sprinkle on the salt and taste as you go. If you have gone overboard on the salt, add in more vegetables to balance out the saltiness.

The next step in the dry-salt method is to massage and squeeze the vegetables. Let the salted vegetables sit for a few minutes before working them, because the salts are starting to work on your behalf, softening the vegetables as the salt pulls the water out. With clean hands, begin to massage the vegetables. The bruising of the vegetables releases their own juices until there is enough liquid to submerge the contents. If the liquid is not enough to submerge the vegetables, water can be added. At this stage experiment with your vegetables by adding in some hot chili peppers, ginger, or garlic.

Brine method

Brining is when kraut is soaked in a solution of water and salt, known as the brine. Soaking vegetables in brine is done for a few hours at a time. If the mixture is saltier, less soaking time is needed. If the mixture is less salty, the vegetables usually soak for a longer period.

Pack it up and ferment

In a stone crock, glass bowl, or glass jar tightly pack in the contents, releasing air pockets. Place a weight such as a plate, a bowl, or a jar to weigh down the kraut until the juices rise above it. If using a wide mouth jar, I often fill a tall, slender glass with water as a weight to place on the vegetables until the juices rise above the vegetables. Leave out at room temperature and out of direct sunlight. Cover contents with a breathable towel to keep debris out. Some cultures lid their ferments and others do not. I'll usually leave the lids off until the fermenting process is complete. Fermenting can be as little as a few hours to a couple weeks or longer. Like all other variations of live food cultures, the fermenting times range from culture to culture as well as personal preference in the sourness and tartness desired. When the desired taste is reached, lid and refrigerate for about two months.[7]

FERMENTED VEGETABLE RECIPES

PICKLED CARROTS WITH GARLIC (BRINE METHOD)

- » 2 cups water
- » 1 Tbsp. sea salt
- » 4 cups thinly sliced or grated carrots (about 5 medium-sized carrots)
- » 2 garlic cloves, crushed

In a glass jar combine the salt and water. Shake to dissolve the salt. Add in remaining ingredients, making sure the brine covers all the vegetables. Set out for at least one day or up to two weeks. Do not drain; leave the vegetables in the brine. Lid and refrigerator in a sealed container for up to two months.

Fills about one quart jar.

Note: The average ratio of salt to water for a brine is 1 Tbsp. salt to 1 cup water. For this recipe, I use much less. To make sure the brine covers the vegetables, place a narrow glass jar on top of the vegetables to allow the juices to rise. Place the jar on a plate as the liquid may rise and spill over.

RED CABBAGE KRAUT (BRINE METHOD)

- » 12 cups water
- » 1 cup sea salt
- » 1 red cabbage (about 4–5 lb.)

Mix the water and salt into a big bowl. Stir the mixture until the salt crystals are dissolved. Cut the cabbage crossways into 2-inch slices. Place the cabbage in a large bowl in the brine with a weight on top to submerse the cabbage. Soak the cabbage in the brine for three to four hours. Drain the cabbage. Do not rinse. Pack the contents into a glass jar, leaving some room at the top. Place the sealed jar in the refrigerator. Refrigerate it up to two months or longer.

Fills a half-gallon jar.

RED VEGETABLE KRAUT (DRY-SALT METHOD)

» 1 red cabbage (about 4–5 lb.)
» 1 large beet
» 1 Tbsp. sea salt (or to taste)

With a food processor or by hand, thinly slice the cabbage and beet. In a large bowl, add the vegetable shreds in with the salt and toss the contents so the salt is spread out evenly. With clean hands, massage and squeeze the contents to release the juices. Stuff the vegetables into a glass bowl or glass jar with a weight, ensuring the liquid rises above the vegetables. You may need to add a little water. Cover with a breathable towel and let sit at room temperature and out of direct sunlight for at least three days. Some ferment much longer, up to two weeks. Lid and refrigerate for up to two months.

Fills a half-gallon jar.

WHITE CABBAGE KRAUT (DRY-SALT METHOD)

» 1 head of cabbage (about 4–5 lb.)
» 1 large carrot
» 1 tsp.–1 Tbsp. sea salt (optional, to taste)

With a food processor or by hand, thinly slice the cabbage and carrot. In a large bowl, add the vegetable shreds in with the salt and toss the contents so the salt is spread out evenly. With clean hands, massage and squeeze the contents to release the juices. Stuff the vegetables into a glass bowl or glass jar with a weight on top, ensuring the liquid rises above the vegetables. A little water may need to be added. Cover with a breathable towel and let sit at room temperature and out of direct sunlight for at least five days. Some ferment much longer, up to two weeks. Lid and refrigerate for two months.

Fills a half-gallon jar.

Rejuvelac Basics: Living Water Through Sprouted Grains and Seeds

Rejuvelac is a rich, nutrient-dense living water that's fermented from sprouted grains or seeds. It is one of nature's finest and most powerful probiotics. Store bought probiotics are pricey, and many are surprised that rejuvelac not only costs pennies on the dollar but ranks in superiority in terms of probiotic quality and quantity. I drink rejuvelac like water and replace water with it in many recipes calling for water. Finding rejuvelac for sale in stores is rare, but it can be made at home. It takes about five days to make and is surprisingly easy once you get into the routine.

Rejuvelac is commonly made from soft spring wheat berries (not hard red winter wheat), barley, rice, buckwheat, and rye. Although the wheat berries are not believed to produce gluten in the sprouting and fermenting process, I tend to use buckwheat in classes for those who are extra cautious about anything containing gluten.

The seeds or grains must be raw or they will not sprout.

Rejuvelac has many health benefits. For starters, rejuvelac cleanses still water, removing heavy metals and releasing nutrients, probiotics, and enzymes. Rejuvelac is rich in vitamins and proteins. The proteins found in rejuvelac are in amino acid form, so they are readily digestible. It also aids the body in superior digestion as it provides the colon with intestinal flora and feeds the healthy bacteria within the colon. All this good bacteria helps our systems fight off bad bacteria.[8] The practice of drinking rejuvelac for its healing properties was popularized by Ann Wigmore, founder of the Ann Wigmore Institute. Ann's teachings and practices have brought countless cancer and diseased patients back to health through rejuvelac and wheatgrass juices.

You can use rejuvelac in place of any recipe calling for water. If the rejuvelac is heated under high temperatures, many of its healing properties will be destroyed; however, it still has mineral and hydration benefits. Rejuvelac is also a starter used in fermented creams, yogurts, and cheeses. Many who understand the healing properties of rejuvelac drink it straight. Stir in some juice, honey, and ice cubes for refreshing beverage.

MAKING REJUVELAC

Here are the basic steps to make your own rejuvelac:

Soak

In a glass jar or bowl, soak ½ cup buckwheat, or other seeds or grains mentioned, covered in water for eight hours or overnight. Buckwheat, or smaller seeds, can take as little as two hours. Keep on the counter and lid the jar with a fine mesh strainer or cover the jar with a breathable cloth. Keep it out of direct sunlight. The grains will start to expand.

Sprout

Drain off the water. Give the grains a good rinse. Do this twice a day (or more) for up to two days or until ⅛-inch little white tails emerge. Draining and rinsing can be done with a bowl and fine mesh strainer, but I prefer using a glass jar with a metal sprouting screen lid for ease and convenience. Plastic sprouting screen lids are also available. Make sure to cover the sprouts with a breathable cloth to keep debris out. Tilt the jar at a 45 degree angle to get more oxygen dispersed to each seed, and let the water drain out.

Ferment

After the berries have sprouted, give them a final rinse and fill the jar with water. There should be approximately 4 to 6 times more water than sprouts. Because the sprouts will have increased in size, the ratio will be 1 cup sprouts to 4 to 6 cups water. Let it sit thirty-six to forty-eight hours. Less time is needed if the weather is warm and more if the weather is cool.

Harvest

Harvest the first batch of rejuvelac. The liquid will be cloudy with a little foam on top—do not be alarmed, this is supposed to happen. Sample the liquid. A slightly sour and fizzy taste should be the result. (If it tastes like it's gone bad or tastes spoiled, discard the batch—you can water your plants with it—and begin again.) This is the first harvest and the strongest flavor. Lid and store the rejuvelac in the refrigerator for up to one month.

Make second and third batches

After the first batch of rejuvelac is harvested, refill the jar of sprouts with the same amount of water for a second and then third batch. The second and third batches need to ferment for only twenty-four hours. After the last batch, discard the sprouted grains or seeds.

RECIPES WITH REJUVELAC

REJUVELAC DRINK

> » 2 cups rejuvelac
> » ½ cup fruit juice
> » 2 Tbsp. lemon juice
> » 3–5 drops stevia
> » 1 cup ice cubes (optional)

Combine, stir, and enjoy!
  With ice, makes about three cups.

SPROUTED BUCKWHEAT MILK

> » 1 cup buckwheat seeds (groats)
> » 2 cups water
> » 2 Tbsp. honey or liquid sweetener

First, sprout the buckwheat (step one of the rejuvelac process). The original one cup of seeds will double in size.

Then rinse and drain. Add water and honey, and blend. Strain the mixture using a nut milk bag. Save this pulp for recipes asking for nut or seed pulps. (I put it into the freezer if I don't have a plan to use it.) The milk stores for up to five days. Blend or shake well before serving.

Drink this fresh or add to smoothies or recipes calling for milk.

Makes over 2 cups.

Note: Simply soaking the seeds for two to eight hours, draining and rinsing, without the little white tails showing, and then making this seed milk works. This is a very healthy milk. While not all will like the flavor for drinking, it is good to use in shakes, smoothies, or any other recipes calling for milk.

While I blend the fresh sprouts with water to make this creamy, mineral-packed, and enzymatic milk, some may take this recipe a step further to make rejuvelac by combining the sprouts and water and leaving it to ferment on the counter for a couple of days before blending and then straining. This is another form of rejuvelac, and is slightly different from the whole berry method previously detailed. For one thing, the whole berry method produces three batches, while this only produces one.

My dad, George, recalls his grandfather having myasthenia gravis, a condition where muscles weaken and get tired. My great-grandmother blended my great-grandfather's food so using his jaw muscles to chew would not be such a chore. George remembers his grandmother sprouting grains on a wet towel and then blending those sprouts with vegetable juices or other liquids. Just like this sprouted milk from buckwheat, those sprouted seeds and grains provide a high mineral content and are loaded with enzymes.

BASIC NUT AND SEED MILKS USING REJUVELAC

Nut and seed milks are creamy, nutritious beverages. Used in smoothies, sauces, soups, and desserts, these creamy liquids are perfect for anyone desiring a nutritional boost or searching for a nondairy replacement. Keep a stash of your favorite nuts and seeds in the pantry to make these milks in no time. While traditionally nut milks involve a blending and straining process of nuts and water, this section allows for the option of replacing the water with rejuvelac. The benefit of course is more probiotics and enzymes. Probiotic milks may achieve a soured or fermented taste when left to ferment.

Most of the time nut and seed milks are drunk the same day they are made, but they can be stored in the refrigerator for up to two days. When stored, give them a good shake or swirl in the blender before drinking because separation will occur. In addition, these milks can be frozen in ice cube trays and then transferred to an airtight container for later use in smoothies and milkshakes. I provide some favorite nut and seed milk recipes in this book, but the following guidelines allow you to create your own so you don't rely on recipes alone. Here are the steps for making nut or seed milk using rejuvelac:

Soaking

Soak nuts or seeds in water, drain, and rinse.

Soaking starts the germination process, releasing tannins and neutralizing enzyme inhibitors. Soaking not only allows the body to better absorb nutrients, it also tones down any bitterness in the nut or seed. The soaking time depends on size. For example, almonds need eight to twelve hours soaking time while sunflower and pumpkin seeds need only two to four hours. Discard the acidic and tinted soaking water. I admit I'm not one to use a chart or timer. I often soak my nuts and seeds overnight, no matter the size, in a cool place or in the refrigerator. There are also times when I forget to soak my nuts or seeds, and I'll soak them for just a few minutes before using. If they soak longer than the allotted time, drain, rinse, and replace the soaking water with fresh water at least once a day for no more than two days, and place them in the refrigerator.

Blending

Blend the nuts or seeds with rejuvelac (or water) to form a thick mixture. Blend in a favorite sweetener, such as a spoonful of honey or maple syrup. A few drops of stevia or a couple pitted dates are also good choices.

The ratio of nuts and seeds to water depends on the creaminess and thickness desired. There are different consistencies: regular and cream. For regular, use one part nuts or seeds to three or four parts rejuvelac (or pure water). For cream, use one part nuts or seeds to two parts rejuvelac (or pure water).

Straining

Pour the liquid mixture into a bowl lined with a nut milk bag or cheesecloth. With one hand holding the top of the bag, use the other hand to gently squeeze from the bottom, allowing the liquid to fill the bowl.

For the probiotic milks or creams, let it sit six to eight hours to ferment. Probiotic milk will have a tartness, but it will not reach the thick consistency of traditionally pasteurized yogurt.

When I first started making nut and seed milks, I used a clean, white T-shirt as a mesh strainer. Living overseas, this invention was birthed out of necessity. A Chinese mesh cloth, used for steaming buns in bamboo baskets or making tofu, works similarly to cheesecloth. For some creams, such as cashew cream, the straining process is omitted.

Saving pulp

Store the leftover nut and seed pulp in a sealed bag or airtight container in the freezer for up to two months. Thaw the pulp a few hours before using.

Nothing needs to be wasted. The nutritious, leftover pulp can be used as flour in dehydrated, or even traditional, crusts, cookies, and breads. Using the rejuvelac method, a nut cheese can also be made (see below for the Almond Pulp Ricotta recipe).

RECIPES FOR DAIRY ALTERNATIVES
AND DAIRY USING REJUVELAC

ALMOND MILK (WITH PROBIOTICS)

- » 1 cup almonds
- » 3–4 cups rejuvelac (use 3–4 cups water for traditional almond milk)
- » 2 Tbsp. honey (or liquid sweetener or 4–6 drops stevia)
- » 1 tsp. vanilla extract

Soak the almonds for eight to twelve hours, and then drain and rinse them. Blend the almonds with all remaining ingredients until smooth. Strain through a nut milk bag or cheesecloth. Drink immediately or refrigerate in an airtight container for up to two days.

Makes about 2½ cups.

Note: For this recipe, the almonds can be replaced Brazil nuts or pumpkin seeds. Experiment: Also, you can use water instead of rejuvelac, if desired, and add in two probiotic capsules.

Health note: Almonds provide an excellent source of protein and calcium. They are also rich in vitamin E, which aids in the prevention of facial lines and wrinkles.

ONE-MINUTE ALMOND MILK (WITH PROBIOTICS)

- » 2 cups rejuvelac (or 2 cups water)
- » ¼ cup almond butter
- » 1 Tbsp. + 1 tsp. honey (or liquid sweetener or 2–4 drops stevia)
- » ½ tsp. vanilla extract

Blend all ingredients together until smooth. Drink immediately or refrigerate in an airtight container for up to two days. Shake well before drinking.

Makes just over 2 cups.

Note: You can replace the rejuvelac with water and add two capsules of probiotic powder. You can also replace the almond butter for another nut or seed butter, such as cashew butter or sunflower seed butter. You can use water instead of rejuvelac, if desired.

ALMOND CREAM (WITH PROBIOTICS)

- » 2 cups almonds
- » 3½ cups rejuvelac (or water)
- » 2 Tbsp. maple syrup or liquid sweetener
- » 1 tsp. vanilla extract

Soak the almonds for eight hours, and then drain and rinse them. Blend the almonds with remaining ingredients until smooth. Strain through a nut milk bag or cheesecloth. Drink immediately or refrigerate in an airtight container for up to two days.

Makes about 3 cups.

Note: Rejuvelac can be replaced with water and two probiotics capsules.

ALMOND YOGURT DRINK (NONDAIRY)

- » 2 cups Almond Cream (with probiotics)
- » ½ tsp. probiotic powder (or 3 capsules)
- » 2 Tbsp. honey or liquid sweetener
- » 2 Tbsp. lemon juice

Place contents in a glass jar and stir contents together with wooden spoon. Leave out at room temperature for eight to twelve hours.

Drink immediately or store in the refrigerator up to five days. Stir or blend before serving.

Makes 2 cups.

Note: The probiotic powder or capsules are important if rejuvelac is not used to make the Almond Cream recipe. Even if you do use rejuvelac in the Almond Cream recipe, adding more probiotics won't hurt. You can also use other types of nut or seed cream in this recipe. This is great to drink alone, to add as the liquid to smoothies, or with cereal or even berries!

PUMPKIN SEED MILK (WITH PROBIOTICS)

- » 1 cup pumpkin seeds
- » 3 cups rejuvelac
- » 2 Tbsp. honey or liquid sweetener
- » 1 tsp. vanilla extract

Soak the pumpkin seeds for four to six hours, and then drain and rinse them. Blend pumpkin seeds and rejuvelac until smooth. Strain through a nut milk bag or cheesecloth. Pour into a glass jar, cover with a breathable cloth, and set on the counter out of direct sunlight for eight to twelve hours. Blend in the remaining ingredients.

Drink immediately or lid and refrigerate for up to two days. Shake well before serving.

Makes about 3 cups.

Note: Rejuvelac can be replaced with water and two probiotics capsules.

ALMOND PULP RICOTTA

» 1½ cups almond pulp (leftover from Almond Milk or Almond Cream recipes)
» 1 Tbsp. olive oil
» ½ tsp. salt (optional or to taste)
» ⅛ tsp. white pepper (optional)

Once you have made the Almond Milk or Cream, leave the pulp in the nut milk bag and set in a strainer on a plate or directly on a plate on the countertop for two to four hours. Then place a weight such as a glass bowl or jar on top so the extra juices can drain out. Let it sit for eight hours or overnight. Drain away excess liquid. Add in the remaining ingredients, adjusting the amount more or less depending on the amount of almond pulp used. Store it in an airtight container in the refrigerator for up to five days.

Makes 1½ cups.

CASHEW SOUR CREAM (NONDAIRY)

» 2 cups cashews
» ¾ cup rejuvelac
» 2 Tbsp. lemon juice
» 1 Tbsp. miso
» ¼ tsp. sea salt
» 1 Tbsp. finely diced chives

Soak the cashews for two hours, and then drain and rinse them. Blend the cashews and rejuvelac until smooth. Blend in the remaining ingredients (except for the chives) and then pour the mixture into a glass bowl or jar. This recipe can be served immediately or fermented. To ferment, cover the sour cream with a breathable towel and let it sit for eight to sixteen hours at room temperature and out of direct sunlight. Refrigerate in an airtight container up to five days. Before serving, garnish with finely diced chives.

Makes about 2 cups.

Note: You may replace the rejuvelac with water.

Salt

If you are trying to cut back on salt, you don't have to use the exact measurements given in the recipes. Cut out a little and see how it tastes.

CASHEW CHEESE ROUND

- » 2 cups cashews
- » ¾ cup rejuvelac
- » 1 Tbsp. lemon juice
- » 2 Tbsp. miso
- » ¼ tsp. sea salt
- » ½ tsp. onion powder
- » ¼ tsp. white pepper
- » ¼ cup maca powder (or almond flour, coconut flour, etc.)

Soak the cashews for two hours, and then drain and rinse them. Blend the cashews, rejuvelac, lemon juice, miso, and sea salt until smooth, and then pour the mixture into a glass bowl or jar. Depending on the blender, a little more rejuvelac may be needed. You can use a food processor instead of a blender, but it will take more time.

Leave the mixture to ferment for twenty to twenty-four hours, folding over the contents with a spatula once or twice in between. Transfer it to a shallow bowl or plate, cover with a breathable towel, nut milk bag, or colander, and move to the refrigerator for three to five days to dry out, folding the contents with a rubber or wooden spatula once a day to help dry out the mixture. Add in the onion powder and white pepper, and add salt to taste. Take the mixture and shape into an oval-shaped ball, roll in ¼ cup maca powder (or almond or coconut flour, etc.), and wrap in a cheesecloth. Set the wrapped cheese ball back in the refrigerator as it will continue to cure and dry out for three days and up to two weeks. You can tell by holding it every now and then. It will feel a little bit harder as the days pass. Once unwrapped from the cheesecloth, store in the refrigerator in an airtight container up to two weeks.

Makes about 1 pound cheese round.

Note: You may replace the rejuvelac with water and add 2 probiotic capsules. You may replace onion powder with garlic powder if preferred.

YOGURT DRINK (DAIRY)

When I was growing up, my dad would bring home raw, unpasteurized milk from neighbors and friends who had cows and goats. Through the years my dairy intake moved to consuming pasteurized, non-organic milk products. When I limited these conventional dairy products in my diet, I noticed a huge difference in my health.

Today I'll have small portions of dairy in organic, unpasteurized (raw), and fermented forms. It's hard to find all three aspects: unpasteurized, organic, and fermented. Buy the raw, organic dairy and then ferment it at home. I keep it in its raw state and ferment it just like I would raw vegetables. Eating fermented dairy is safe, and the healthy benefit of all the good bacteria and probiotics makes it worth the extra step.

» 2 cups raw, unpasteurized milk (or cream for a thicker consistency)
» ½ tsp. probiotic powder (or 3 probiotic capsules)
» 2 Tbsp. lemon juice
» 2 Tbsp. raw honey or liquid sweetener

Put ingredients into a glass jar. Stir ingredients, but don't overstir or shake the jar to prevent pre-curdling. Cover with a breathable cloth. Leave alone and let sit at room temperature and out of direct sunlight for eight hours or overnight. As the jar sits still, the mixture will gel into a yogurt. Lid and refrigerate in an airtight container up to five days. Stir before serving.

Makes just over 2 cups.

Note: You can replace the milk or cream with a nut or seed milk or cream. I know you may be nervous about leaving dairy at room temperature for so long. You can make this same recipe and refrigerate for eight to twelve hours, instead. Raw milk is banned in some states, so you may have difficulty finding it. Also, this does not thicken in the same way as traditional yogurt. However, it still tastes good as a drink, in smoothies, and with granola.

Sour Cream (dairy)

- » 1 cup raw, unpasteurized cream (goat or cow)
- » 1 Tbsp. apple cider vinegar or lemon juice
- » 1 Tbsp. miso paste
- » ½ tsp. probiotic powder (or 3 probiotic capsules)
- » Pinch of salt (optional or to taste)

Put ingredients into a glass jar and stir with wooden spoon. Don't overstir or shake the jar to prevent pre-curdling. Cover with a breathable cloth. Leave alone and let it sit at room temperature and out of direct sunlight for eight hours or overnight. Instead, as the jar sits still, it will gel into a sour cream consistency. Lid and refrigerate in an airtight container up to five days.

Makes just over 1 cup.

Note: Although this is not as thick as store-bought sour cream, it is still great as a salad dressing or dip or with chili or soup.

Fermenting Dairy Products

Leaving dairy products out at room temperature scares most people. Traditionally milks just sat out at room temperature without a starter and would start to clabber, turning into a thickened mud or gel through the fermenting process. However, the key in these recipes is that the milks and creams are unpasteurized, in a raw state. Many recipes call for either lemon juice, white vinegar, or a probiotic. I like to use a combo of a probiotic and lemon, or a probiotic and apple cider vinegar (for the extra nutrients and to get those probiotics generating quickly).[9]

Seed G-raw-nola (nut and gluten free)

I love this Seed G-raw-nola with any milk, but especially with yogurt, drizzled with raw honey, and topped with a few fresh berries. This makes a good breakfast, meal, or even dessert!

» 1 cup pumpkin seeds
» 1 cup sunflower seeds
» 1 cup raisins
» ¼ cup sesame seeds
» 2 Tbsp. ground flaxseed

Combine all ingredients in a food processor. Pulse until the seeds are broken up into two or three pieces.

Makes over 3 cups.

CHAPTER 6

Get Juiced: From Pulp Fiction to Pulp Kitchen

ODAY'S FOUNTAIN OF Youth" really should be another name for a juice machine. From preventing disease to recovering from disease, reversing the clock, building the immune system, or fighting off fatigue, wrinkles, and the aging process, juicing is where it's at.[1] I once read that the question was not "To juice or not to juice?" but rather, "How many times per day should one juice?" Eating raw fruits and vegetables—blended or whole—is a nutritious way to get fiber and nutrients. With juicing, however, there is a higher concentration and higher absorbable amounts of nutrients, such as phytonutrients and antioxidants, with less fiber.

There are different quality juicers at different prices. I've used several different types of juicers over the years, some being much better quality than others. The Gerson Therapy has helped cancer and disease patients recover through juicing, so it is well worth the investment in purchasing a good juicer.[2]

Wouldn't it be better to prevent a disease than recover from one? With that said, the best juicer to use is the one you will start using today. Go to your nearest thrift store and you may see a lineup of steeply discounted juice machines reminiscent of enthusiast owners of the past who went on a juicing kick for a month or two only to find the machine gradually getting in the way of other kitchen appliances and collecting dust. Therefore, use the juicer you have or get one within your budget. Then, when you know if you will use it, you can consider purchasing your next upgrade.

While I love the health and beauty benefits of fresh fruit and vegetable juices, juicing at home is one of my biggest struggles. Some mornings, the last thing I have time for is juicing, especially cleaning out the juice machine. Because I find this such a challenge, I added to my morning routine: "Drink Fresh Juice."

When I juice, I try to juice as much as I can, sometimes double the juice recipes provided in this book, so they last longer and over a two- or three-day period. While fresh juices are the most beneficial when drunk immediately after juicing, I've had to pick my battles, spending less time in the kitchen juicing and making my juice last longer, as well as going to the local natural foods store to pick up freshly made juice.

The juice recipes provide one or two servings, each recipe filling about a quart-size jar. However, this will depend on the size and amount of each type of produce juiced, as well as the different water content of each type of produce.

Here is some information on the types of juicers available:

- **Centrifugal Juicers:** The benefit of centrifugal juicers is that they are fast, efficient, and easy to use. They work by pushing the fruits and vegetables through a rotating disc as the pulp is strained through a screen. Centrifugal juicers are the most affordable. The downside to these types of juicers is they leave quite a bit of pulp, especially with leafy greens. On the cool side, I found that by juicing kale leaves with stems, I had a wonderful amount of finely chopped kale in the pulp compartment of the juicer. This went right into salads with no extra chopping necessary. If you are just starting out, a centrifugal juicer is a good way to go.

- **Masticating Juicers:** Masticating juicers have a single rotating gear. I liken it to a cow slowly chewing its cud; a masticating juicer chomps the fruits and vegetables, squeezing the juices outs. The benefits of masticating juicer are their efficiency with the juice quantity being maximized and the leftover pulp being drier than a centrifugal juicer. Because these juicers run at slow speeds using less heat, there is less oxidization.

- **Tribulating Juicers:** Tribulators or twin-gear juicers are top-of-the-line. The two gears rotate inward, grinding the fruits and vegetables at low speeds and then using a hydraulic press for juice extraction. The result produces a very dry pulp with no heat. Research shows this type of juicer produces up to fifty-percent higher nutrient content. This is the type of juicer recommended for the Gerson Therapy. Although it is significantly more expensive, your regained health is a priceless return on investment.[3]

While it's better to drink fresh juice quickly to preserve all the living goodness, I often make extra and store it in glass jars in the refrigerator for the next couple of days. I just don't like cleaning a juicer more than once a day. If you want to drink fresh juice three or more times a day, go for it! You could do a combination of juicing once per day and then picking up your juice order at your local co-op. Call a day or more in advance, and I'm sure you can work something out on a weekly basis. I admit I've fallen off the bandwagon on juicing many times. Just like returning to the gym, once I am back into juicing, I wonder how could I live without it. How could I live without nature's life-giving, nutrient-packed, and enzyme-rich gift? Get into a routine, follow these tips, and start juicing today!

TIPS FOR JUICING

Follow these tips to make the juicing process easier:

- Keep a scrap bin for juicing in the refrigerator. All the odds and ends of chopped produce from recipes you have made can add up. The day before you go produce shopping, juice everything in the bin and start over.

- Wash and bag your vegetables the night before. If you are going to juice two or more times per day, have a bag of ready-to-juice items in each bag.

- I use clean pillowcases to wrap and store washed produce. I learned this from a client of Armenian heritage who wrapped her washed produce in these cotton pouches about half the size of a pillowcase. It works well to keep produce fresh and dry, soaking up excess moisture and allowing the produce to breath. Storing produce in brown paper bags or paper towels also works well.

- If you are serious about your juicing regimen but lack the time, consider juicing once per day and jarring the rest for later. Due to oxidization, drinking juice immediately after juicing is best.

- Join a CSA (community-supported agriculture) that has seasonal produce delivered straight to your door. This saves time and is a great way to support local farmers.

- After your juicer is washed and dried, quickly reassemble it. Waking up in the morning to your juicer disassembled in bits and pieces may discourage you from juicing. A fully assembled juicer in the morning says, "Let's juice!"

Tips for Using Leftover Pulp

Returning your juice pulp to the garden compost pile is good for putting nourishment back into the soil. However, you can also use the pulp in some instances. Here are a few tips on using your pulp:

- Add a cup or two of vegetable-based pulp to the blended soups in this book, or use it to thicken your own homemade sauces and soups

- Add a cup or two of fruit-based pulp to your homemade muffins and breads

- Feed it to your animals and pets

- Use cucumber pulp for face masks

REGENERATION YOUTH MASK

A spa I went to in Shanghai had a cucumber mask, and I was almost positive it was the leftover pulp from their cucumber juices. It's a great idea! Here is a facial recipe I've made with cucumber and other pulps. If the cucumber is mixed with other fruits and greens, it's fine, like a multi-mineral pack for the face!

This mask wakes up skin as nutrients are absorbed though the pores. Whether eaten or applied externally, cucumbers are a classic beauty food for the skin.

» 1 cup cucumber pulp
» 1 Tbsp. lemon juice
» 1 Tbsp. honey
» 1 Tbsp. bentonite clay

Mix all ingredients together. Apply the mixture or store in the refrigerator up to five days.

A chilled mask is extra refreshing and invigorates facial tissues. If the pulp is stored in the freezer, store about ¼ cup amounts in little plastic bags and transfer them to the refrigerator the night before using them. Place a few in the refrigerator at a time so they are ready to use when you need them. Leave the mask on for ten minutes or longer and rinse.

JUICE RECIPES: GREENER-BASED-GREEN LIKE YOU'VE NEVER SEEN

CABBAGE PATCH

- » 1 head cabbage (1 lb.)
- » 2 pears
- » 1 lime, peeled

Juice it! Drink up.

Serves 1–2.

Health note: Reduce inflammation with cabbage and lemons. This juice will help relieve constipation and is a digestion regulator. The rich sulfur content in cabbage makes it a trademark for nourishing skin to beauty and radiance. It also contains vitamin U, a remedy for ulcers.[4]

GREEN GARDEN

- » 1 bunch collard greens (1 lb.)
- » 4–6 celery stalks
- » 1 large cucumber or zucchini
- » 2 green apples (optional)
- » 2–4 sprigs basil, cilantro, or parsley

Juice it! Drink up.

Serves 1–2.

Health note: Leafy greens and cucumber peel are known for their rich, skin-enriching sulfur content. Collard greens are a chlorophyll-rich food and useful to cleanse the liver of excess and stagnancy.[5]

A Fix for Overeating

I love celery, it has the perfect crunch. If you are find yourself overeating, try eating a couple stalks of celery in between or during meals.

GREEN SUPREME

- » 1 head broccoli (1 lb.)
- » 1 bunch or big handful spinach
- » 2 celery stalks
- » 2 green apples or pears

Juice it! Drink up.

Serves 1–2.

Health note: This disease fighter and inflammation preventer is like putting a miracle IV into your bloodstream. The greener your juice, the more phytonutrients and chlorophyll it has. Broccoli contains more vitamin C than citrus. Spinach is an excellent source of calcium.

In addition to its rich mineral content, broccoli is one of the best sources of beta carotene, which is a powerful anti-carcinogen, specifically pointing to fighting colon, stomach, and esophageal cancers.[6]

THE GREEN RIND

- » 1–2 lb. green rinds from watermelon
- » 1 lime, peeled
- » Pinch sea salt (optional)

Juice it! Drink up.

Serves 1–2.

Health note: Watermelon is often used to cleanse and restore kidney health. Using watermelon rind is a low sugar way to do the same thing, but with the added nourishment from the rinds, which hydrates and restores the skin as well. Nothing needs to be wasted. This is one of my favorite juices, mainly because I used to just toss the rinds out. Now I appreciate all these beautifying liquids. Before throwing your watermelon rinds to the compost pile, juice them. This lightly sweetened juice is one of my favorite skin quenchers. I'll juice as much as I can, drink a glass, and then put the rest in a jar and bring with me.

KALER CUCUMBER COMBO

- » 1 bunch kale (1 lb.)
- » 2 large cucumbers

» 2 pears or apples
» 1 lemon, peeled

Juice it! Drink up.

Serves 1–2.

Health note: Cucumbers are wonderful skin cleansers as well as bloating and swelling preventers. The leftover pulp can be refrigerated for up to three days and used as a face mask to reduce swelling.

KALE STEM JUICE

» 20 or more kale stems (or stalks with leaves OK) (about 1 lb.)
» 4 green apples or pears

Juice it! Drink up.

Serves 1–2.

Note: Many recipes call for kale leaves, de-stemming the leaves. So before putting the stems into the garbage or compost, save them in your juicing bin and throw them in with your juice.

Health note: Kale is a relative of cabbage, brussels sprouts, and cauliflower and is in the mustard family. It's one of the most vitamin-rich and mineral-packed leafy greens around, helping to prevent cancer, arthritis, constipation, and bladder problems.[7]

MINTY CLEANSER

» 4 cucumbers (about 1 lb.)
» 2 green apples
» 2–4 mint sprigs

Juice it! Drink up.

Serves 1–2.

Note: This is a cooling toner. This juice has just the right hint of mint. With pungent herbs, just a few sprigs will do. Try replacing the mint with some cilantro, basil, or parsley. The leftover minty pulp can be refrigerated for up to three days and used as a face mask to reduce swelling.

Health note: The malic and tartaric acids in apples inhibit growth of bad bacteria in the digestive tract. The pectin in apples also works as a detoxifier for residues in radiation and heavy metals, such as mercury.[8]

PEARED WITH ZUCCHINI

Zucchini abounds in the summer! My dad says there are two reasons to lock your car at church in the summer. One is to prevent theft, and the other is to keep people from gifting you with zucchini. No more fears about what to do with this wonderful squash because we can juice it!

» 2–4 large zucchini (1 or 2 lb.)
» 2 pears
» 2–4 sprigs basil

Juice it! Drink up.

Serves 1–2.

Health note: This juice helps with constipation, gallbladder issues, and inflammation. In the summer months when zucchini abounds, juice! Zucchini is high in vitamin C and lutein for eye health.[9]

ROMAINE CALM AND TURNIP THE BEET

» 1 head romaine lettuce
» 2 small beetroots (stems optional)
» 1 apple
» 1-inch cubed turnip

Juice it! Drink up.

Serves 1–2.

Health note: This is a liver detoxifier and circulation booster. Beets are another silicon-rich vegetable with deep-cleansing properties, cleansing the blood and liver. This juice improves circulation and the small amount of turnip gives a surprising amount of edginess.

I'LL BE BOK CHOY

» 2 lb. bok choy
» 2 large cucumbers
» 2 green apples
» 1-inch cube ginger or turmeric or 1 clove garlic

Juice it! Drink up.

Serves 1–2.

Health note: This is a great liver cleanser and inflammation regulator. The leftover pulp can be refrigerated for up to three days and used as a face mask to reduce swelling.

Fruitier Based—Just Showing My Sweet Side

Citrus Regenerator

» 2 grapefruits
» 2 oranges
» 1 lemon
» 1 lime
» 1-inch cubed ginger

Juice it! Drink up.

Serves 1–2.

Health note: This juice is full of antioxidants. Citrus fruits are age-fighters and circulation boosters. To reduce your waste, you can take the sliced citrus peels and a slice of ginger and pour hot water over them for a cleansing morning tea.

Enzyme Repairer

» ½ or more pineapple
» 2 cucumbers or zucchini
» 4 lemons
» 1 bunch parsley

Juice it! Drink up.

Serves 1–2.

Health note: Pineapple contains the enzyme bromelain, and in more concentrated amounts in the fruit's core. (I either juice the center or chew on it as a snack.) This juice is packed with vitamin C. Lemons are antiseptic and anti-microbial, fighting off infections and building the liver.[10]

For the Love of Beet

» 2–4 beetroots (stems optional)
» 2 pears
» 1 medium zucchini
» 1 lemon

Juice it! Drink up.

Serves 1–2.

Health note: This is a liver regenerator and it also relieves constipation. Beets are another silicon-rich vegetable with deep-cleansing properties, cleansing the blood and liver and improving circulation.[11] Be forewarned that if you start consuming high amounts of beets, your urine may turn red. This can be scary for some, especially those who think it's blood. However, it's just a reminder that the red goodness in beets is cleansing your blood and liver.

Ginger-Spiked Watermelon

» 1 medium watermelon
» 1-inch cube ginger

Juice it! Drink up.

Serves 1–2.

Health note: This is a kidney flusher with a circulation boost of ginger to stay invigorated throughout the day. When juicing watermelon, juice the rind as well.

Grape Expectations

» 1 large cluster grapes
» 2 large cucumbers or zucchini
» 1 beetroot

Juice it! Drink up.

Serves 1–2.

Health note: This is full of antioxidants and is a liver detoxifier. To lessen the sweetness of this juice, add a cucumber or zucchini. You can also take this juice and mix in a one-to-one ratio of rejuvelac (see chapter 5 for more info).

IDAHO JUICE

> » 3–4 large potatoes (1 lb.)
> » 1 jicama root (1 lb.)

Juice it! Drink up.

Serves 1–2.

Note: Finding organically grown fruit year round is tough, but this two-ingredient juice is sweetened with the jicama. It's quite simple and refreshing.

Health note: A potato has a high amount of vitamin C, ranking just below citrus fruits; however, it must be raw.[12] Potatoes also reduce inflammation and treat ulcers. Drunk fresh, potato juice has antibiotic properties establishing healthy gut flora in the intestines.[13]

Raw Potatoes

Who says you cannot eat a potato raw? Potatoes are high in potassium, and they relieve inflammation and lower blood pressure.[14] I get my potatoes at the local organic market. (I mention this because potatoes are now becoming GMO, genetically modified, so organic is especially key here.)

PINEAPPLE COLADA

> » 1 pineapple
> » 4 stalks celery
> » 1 orange
> » 1 lemon
> » 1 lime

Juice it! Drink up.

Serves 1–2.

Note: The celery in this colada adds a savory hint. For a creamy colada, add a half cup of your favorite milk, cream, or yogurt and shake before drinking.

Health note: The enzyme bromelain, in more concentrated forms in the pineapple's core, increases the body's digestive ability to fight against worms. Pineapples treats indigestion and constipation.[15]

Sweet Greens

» 3 apples
» 2 kale leaves with stem
» 2 celery stalks
» 1-inch cubed onion or 1 clove garlic

Juice it! Drink up.

Serves 1–2.

Health note: The pectin in apples aids in digestion and also removes cholesterol, toxic metals such as lead and mercury, and residues of radiation from the system. Adding a hint of garlic or onion is surprisingly tasty and a reminder of the antioxidant and cleansing effects it has.[16]

Sweet Potato and Carrot

» 2 medium-sized sweet potatoes or yams
» 2 large carrots
» 2 oranges
» Pinch cinnamon (optional)

Juice it! Drink up.

Serves 1–2.

Health note: Carrots fight cancer, clear up acne, relieve constipation, and give skin a glow.[17] Sweet potatoes and yams reduce inflammation. They can also help your kidneys, spleen, and pancreas. This vitamin A booster is a strong detoxifier as well, and it alkalizes the body and nourishes for healthy and radiant skin tone.[18]

Juice Scraps

» 1 scrap bin worth of produce
» 1 new shopping list for the next juice

Juice it! Drink up.

Detox Delish

Note: This is a regenerator of all things good and it ensures nothing is wasted. Keep a tub in the fridge labeled "Juice Scraps" or "Juice Bin."

FRESH-DRINK RECIPES

BERRY FRESH INFUSION

» 4 cups water, rejuvelac, or coconut water
» ½ cup blueberries
» ½ cup raspberries
» 1 lemon, sliced

Fill a quart-size glass jar with ingredients and place in the refrigerator for a few hours or overnight so the ingredients can fuse. Straining is optional. The fruit in the water makes a nice presentation when serving in a pitcher or glass.

Makes 4 cups.

Note: This is a refreshing quencher with antioxidants and vitamins. Add a bit of stevia or honey to taste if preferred. Juice or compost the remaining contents.

CHIA FRUIT DRINK

» ½ cup warm water
» ¼ cup chia seeds
» 2 cups fresh juice mixtures (use one of the three options below)

Green Apple-Lime

» 4 green apples
» 1 lime, peeled

Grape-Beet

» 2 bunches grapes
» 1 small beetroot

Orange-Ginger

» 4 large oranges
» 1–2-inch ginger, sliced

Juice one of the combinations of produce. In a glass jar add chia seeds and juice to water. Cover it and shake well. Let sit for twenty minutes on the counter or overnight in the refrigerator. It can be stored in the refrigerator for a couple days.

Makes 3 cups.

Health note: Chia is a good source of protein. It's a complete protein, containing all the amino acids needed as well as omega-3 fatty acids.

CULTURED CABBAGE JUICE (PROBIOTIC)

» ½ cabbage, chopped
» 4–5 cups water
» ¼–½ tsp. sea salt

Use a food processor or blender to chop the cabbage. If you use a blender, pulse the mixture so it is still lumpy. Blend all the ingredients together. In a half-gallon jar or two one-quart glass jars pour the mixture in, leaving an inch or two of room at the top. Place in a cool place and out of direct sunlight for at least three days and up to one week, agitating the jar daily. If the cabbage is smooth rather than lumpy, cut back on the amount of time it is left to ferment. After day three, taste daily until the desired tartness is reached. Strain the liquid. Lid and store in the refrigerator up to two weeks.

Fills a half-gallon jar.

Note: Commonly referred to as cultured cabbage juice, this beverage can be served with any meal or drunk alone.[19]

GREEN LIGHT INFUSION

» 4 cups water, rejuvelac, or coconut water
» 1 lime, sliced (with peel)
» 1 cucumber, sliced
» 2 mint sprigs

Fill a quart-size glass jar with ingredients and place in the refrigerator for a few hours or overnight so the ingredients can fuse.

Makes 4 cups.

Note: This is a refreshing quencher with antioxidants and vitamins. Add a bit of stevia or honey to taste if preferred. Either juice the remaining contents or compost.

MINTY COCONUT HYDRATOR

» 2–3 cups coconut water (or water from one coconut)
» 4–6 mint leaves (peppermint or spearmint)

Blend all ingredients together and strain through a nut milk bag or cheesecloth if desired. Drink immediately.

Serves 1–2.

Note: Try this with a few basil leaves or cilantro for a hint of flavor. Drink throughout the day.

Coconut Water

I love coconut water. I used to take morning walks to a local vendor where I'd buy two coconuts, drink the water from one there and then drink the water from the other one on the walk home. This minty refresher is one of creation's natural electrolyte drinks, hydrating the organs and keeping skin youthful and supple.

REJUVENATING JUICE COMBO

This beverage using a fruit juice of red grapes or beetroot is great for a workout drink and is not overly sweet. It can also quench thirst and replete nutrients after a rigorous gym workout.

» 2 cups rejuvelac
» 2 cups favorite fruit-based juice

Stir and enjoy. Store in sealed glass jar in the refrigerator for up to five days.

Makes 4 cups.

SUPERFOOD "HOT" COCOA

- » 2 cups Almond Milk or Cream (chapter 5)
- » 1 Tbsp. + 1 tsp. honey or liquid sweetener
- » 2 tsp. coconut oil
- » 2 tsp. cacao powder or carob powder
- » 1 Tbsp. hemp hearts (or ½ tsp hemp powder) (optional)
- » 1 tsp. reishi powder (optional)
- » Pinch sea salt

Blend all ingredients together until smooth. Serve at room temperature or heated.
Serves 2.

HERBAL DETOX TEAS

I used to be an avid green tea drinker but found the high amounts of caffeine made me jittery. It's really a personal choice, but I tend to lean towards herbal teas, bought in the bulk tea and herbal section. Steeped in hot water, drink these teas in the morning or late at night before bedtime:

- Alfalfa

- Dandelion flower

- Dandelion root

- Eucalyptus

- Marshmallow root

- Milk thistle

There is a list of detoxifiers that can be added to your tea below. The list below came about in a couple of ways: First, I browse the bulk section of the neighborhood organic co-op and try new things. Second, as I read the ingredients of store-bought and pricey detoxification kits, they often listed these ingredients, which one can buy and enjoy in teas instead of swallowing in supplement form. Here are some detoxifiers I use in tea:

Detox Delish

- Cinnamon
- Goji berries
- Hawthorn berries
- Juniper berries
- Lemon slices
- Lime slices
- Ginger slices
- Turmeric slices

I like to steep both the tea and detox ingredients. Serving these in a see-through coffee press makes a beautiful presentation when serving guests.

CHAPTER 7

Smoothie Operator: Freshen Up With Delicious Blends

A S A CHEF and an instructor teaching private clients and large groups, I've used all types of kitchen appliances. However, the electrical appliance I use the most, hands down, is a blender for its ease and convenience. Starting out I centered most of my class recipes around a household blender. It was simply the best way to show people that eating by blending up delicious recipes can be quick, easy, and healthy. Blenders are easy to clean, and they are also versatile. They blend smoothies, purée soups, crush ice, and grind nuts and seeds.

Blenders normally hold five cups. If I'm home, I will often take advantage of the size of the blender by making enough to have some later in the day. Travel-size blenders also work, but the recipes in this book will need to be divided in half or in proportion to the size of the mini blender used. You might be wondering what type of blender to use. There is a full range of blenders, from conventional household blenders to more expensive commercial, high-speed blenders. Most restaurants and smoothie bars use high-speed blenders. While I prefer a high-speed blender over a conventional blender, the recipes in this book accommodate both types. My suggestion is to start with the blender you have. If contemplating taking out a small loan to buy a commercial blender, start with what you have and work your way up. Remember, the best blender to have is the one you'll start using today!

For the smoothie recipes in this chapter, use the amounts given in each recipe as a guideline as the exact amount of each ingredient may depend on the size of the fruit or the desired sweetness.

Warning!

Smoothies may contain fresh, organic, leafy green vegetables and fruits, which are loaded with nutrients needed for healthy hair, skin, and nails. If signs of improved digestion, improved mental clarity, and increased energy levels result, contact your local farmer for a consultation on the full range of organic produce available. In the case of weight loss or an improved appearance, contact a style consultant immediately for a new wardrobe and makeover. Make a green smoothie now before this offer expires—or you do!

How can a green-colored drink produce die-hard, green- smoothie converts? Popularized by Victoria Boutenko, green smoothies are a combination of leafy greens sweetened with fruits. It's a liquid, power-packed meal. Fruits add a healthy load of carbohydrates, fiber, antioxidants, and nutrients. Likewise, leafy greens are like superior multi-vitamins with minerals and phytonutrients packed into every leaf. The chlorophyll gives leaves their vibrant shades of green through the absorption of sunlight, working as internal healers and cleansers. Most of my classmates and instructors at the culinary institute I attended ate a raw, plant-based diet, and juices and smoothies seemed to be star players in their daily eating regimen.

Although I love leafy greens in salads, I found that in order to increase the amount of greens in my diet, a blended green smoothie or green juice was the way to go. Also, they increased my nutrient intake and improved my digestion. Whether for breakfast, a meal, or a snack, drinking a green smoothie is like sipping the sun's pure energy.

BUILDING BLOCKS FOR MAKING GREEN SMOOTHIES

Green smoothies are often a 60 percent to 40 percent ratio of fruits to leafy greens. They can also be a fifty-fifty ratio of fruits and veggies. Yet, another type of green smoothie is one with almost all greens and half an orange or squeeze of lemon to cut the bitterness of the greens. It must be obvious by now that there are no strict rules for making green smoothies. Nevertheless, there are some guidelines to follow. I provide green smoothie recipes in this book, but put aside your measuring cups and spoons after a while because you are soon going to be your own green smoothie expert!

Here are some basic guidelines to follow when making a green smoothie:

1. *Choose leafy greens:* Choose one, two, or three leafy greens, such as romaine lettuce, kale, and spinach. I tend to choose leafy greens without too much pungency so they don't overpower the fruitiness of the smoothie. Also, alternating the variety of greens offers a broader spectrum of nutrients.

2. *Choose fruits:* Choose one, two, or three fruits, such as oranges, lemons, limes, bananas, mangos, pineapples, blueberries, or raspberries. Think of another fruit? Great! Do avoid melons in smoothies because they digest better eaten alone. Changing fruits from day to day offers a wider range of nutrients.

3. *Add supplements:* This step is optional. In small amounts, add some pungent herbs such as parsley, mint, basil, or cilantro. You can also add powders such as chlorella, spirulina, young wheat grass, and young barley grass. Supplements are good boosters, and are great to bring on trips when eating enough greens is a challenge.

4. *Blend:* Add water or juice to the greens and blend until smooth. Then add the fruits. Most drink green smoothies at room temperature for optimum digestion, but ice cubes can be added. Add any frozen fruit chunks or ice cubes in gradually.

FRUIT- AND VEGETABLE-BASED SMOOTHIES

ENZYME RELEASER

» 2 cups sprouts (broccoli, clover, alfalfa)
» 2 bananas, fresh or frozen
» 2 cups pineapple
» 1–2 cups rejuvelac, coconut water, or water
» 1–2 cups ice cubes (optional)

Blend all ingredients together until smooth, blending the ice cubes last. Drink immediately or store in the refrigerator for a day.

Serves 1–2.

Note: Avoid spicy sprouts so they don't overpower the smoothie. Although this smoothie has a lot of green energy and phytonutrients, it's really not so green looking.

GRAPEFRUIT-GOJI DETOX

» 1 Tbsp. goji berries
» 2 grapefruits
» 2 bananas
» 1–2 cups rejuvelac, coconut water, or water
» 2 cups ice cubes (optional)

Soak the goji berries in the rejuvelac or water for five minutes to soften. Blend all ingredients together until smooth, blending the ice cubes last. Drink immediately or store in the refrigerator for a day.

Serves 1–2.

Note: Citrus juices and smoothies are like giving our skin a spring show of youth. The tartness of the fruits is a reminder that our skin will be thankful for the antioxidants and detox elements that keep our skin supple and radiant.

GREEN MEANS GO

- » 1 big handful kale or collard greens
- » 2 medium mangos
- » 1 cup rejuvelac, coconut water, or water
- » 2 Tbsp. lemon juice
- » 1 tsp. ground flaxseed
- » 1 tsp. bentonite clay
- » 2 cups ice cubes (optional)

Blend all ingredients together until smooth, blending the ice cubes last. Drink immediately or refrigerate for a day.

Serves 1–2.

Note: Adding a bit of flaxseed and clay to any smoothie will thicken it right up, so you may need to add more liquid.

Health note: Flaxseed and clay are colon cleansers.

GREEN APPLE DETOX SMOOTHIE

- » 1 green apple
- » 1 banana, fresh or frozen, sliced
- » 1 cup water, coconut water, or rejuvelac
- » 2 Tbsp. lemon juice
- » 2 Tbsp. apple cider vinegar
- » 1 Tbsp. honey or liquid sweetener
- » 1–2 cups ice cubes (optional)

Blend all ingredients together until smooth, blending the ice cubes last. Drink immediately or store in the refrigerator for a day.

Serves 1–2.

Health note: The pectin in apples helps to both dissolve gallstones and prevent gallstones for gallbladder health.

KALE OR BE KALED

- » 1 handful kale leaves
- » 1 orange
- » 1 banana, fresh or frozen
- » 4 Tbsp. lemon juice
- » 2 cups rejuvelac, coconut water, or water
- » 2 cups ice cubes (optional)

Blend all ingredients together until smooth, blending the ice cubes last. If using a conventional blender, and not a commercial blender, blend the leafy greens with the liquid first until smooth and then add the remaining ingredients. Drink immediately or store in the refrigerator for a day.

Serves 1–2.

Note: For green kale smoothies, I'll de-stem the kale and blend the leaves since the stems are tough. The stems can be thrown into the juice bin and juiced later.

KIWI-SPINACH CLEANSER

Whether for a meal or a snack, this green energy will keep you moving throughout the day. I find a green smoothie as an afternoon snack is exactly what my body needs.

» 1–2 big handfuls spinach
» 3 kiwis
» 1 cup pineapple
» 1 lime, squeezed
» 1 cup rejuvelac, coconut water, or water
» 2 cups ice cubes (optional)

Blend all ingredients together until smooth, blending the ice cubes last. If using a conventional blender and not a commercial blender, blend the leafy greens with the liquid first until smooth and then add the remaining ingredients. Drink immediately or store in the refrigerator for a day.

Serves 1–2.

RED BERRY BANANA

This antioxidant booster is full of berry enzymes.

» ½ cup raspberries
» ½ cup strawberries
» 2 bananas, fresh or frozen
» 2 cups rejuvelac, coconut water, or water
» 2 cups ice cubes (optional)
» 3–5 drops liquid stevia

Blend all ingredients together until smooth, blending the ice cubes last. Drink immediately or refrigerate for a day.

Serves 1–2.

SUMMER SALAD SMOOTHIE

This is a quick energy meal for when you just don't have time to eat a huge salad. While it's difficult to get two or three salads in a day, it is easier to blend them up; we get the same benefit, but the nutrients are more absorbable.

» 2–4 handfuls chopped romaine
» 1 apple, chopped
» 1 mango, cubed
» 4 Tbsp. lemon juice
» 1 Tbsp. sesame seeds
» 1 Tbsp. flaxseed oil
» 2 cups rejuvelac, coconut water, or water
» 2 cups ice cubes (optional)

Blend all ingredients together until smooth, blending the ice cubes last. If using a conventional blender and not a commercial blender, blend the leafy greens with the liquid first until smooth and then add the remaining ingredients. Drink immediately or store in the refrigerator for a day.

Serves 1–2.

Extra Bananas

Never throw away a banana again. The best way to eat bananas is when they are spotted with brown on the outside. You can peel and slice bananas in 1 cup portion amounts to freeze and use in smoothies later. Berries also store well in the freezer.

MILK-BASED BLENDS

4Bs: BUCKWHEAT, BANANAS, BERRIES, AND (NUT) BUTTER

They say everything tastes better with butter, especially with nut and seed butters! That is true for this smoothie.

» 2 cups Sprouted Buckwheat Milk (chapter 5)
» 2 Tbsp. sunflower seed butter
» ½ cup strawberries

» 2 bananas, fresh or frozen
» 1 Tbsp. honey or liquid sweetener
» Pinch sea salt (optional)
» 2 cups ice cubes (optional)

Blend all ingredients together until smooth. Blend the ice cubes last. Drink immediately or refrigerate for a day.

Serves 1–2.

BERRY YOGURT SMOOTHIE

» 1 cup Almond Yogurt Drink or another milk (chapter 5)
» 1 cup rejuvelac, coconut water, or water
» ½ cup raspberries or strawberries
» 1 banana
» 2 Tbsp. honey or liquid sweetener (or 4–6 drops stevia)
» Pinch sea salt (optional)
» 2 cups ice cubes (optional)

Blend all ingredients together until smooth, blending the ice cubes last. Drink immediately or refrigerate for a day.

Serves 1–2.

Note: This smoothie makes a good addition to the Seed G-raw-nola in chapter 5.

CAROB-HEMP PROTEIN SHAKE

» 4–6 dates (honey or medjool), pitted
» 2 cups Almond Milk (or other milk)
» 2 bananas, fresh or frozen
» 1 cup kale leaves (about 1 handful)
» ¼ cup hemp hearts (or 1 tsp. hemp powder)
» 2 Tbsp. almond butter (or nut or seed butter)
» 2 tsp. carob powder
» ½ tsp. vanilla extract
» Pinch cinnamon
» Pinch sea salt (optional)
» 2 cups ice cubes (optional)

Soak the dates in the milk for 15 minutes to soften them. (If the dates are not hard or if you have a commercial blender, you can skip this step.) Blend all ingredients together until smooth, blending the ice cubes last. Drink immediately or store in the refrigerator for a day.

Serves 1–2.

Note: When a recipe calls for cacao powder, I often like to use half carob and cacao. I love the nutrient-rich properties of chocolate, and in combination with the sweet, mineral-rich carob it's a superfood combo that is hard to beat.

MANGO LASSI SMOOTHIE

» 2 cups mangos, fresh or frozen
» 1 cup Almond Yogurt Drink (chapter 5)
» 1 cup rejuvelac, coconut water, or water
» 2 Tbsp. honey or liquid sweetener (or 4–6 drops stevia)
» Pinch sea salt (optional)
» 2 cups ice cubes (optional)

Blend all ingredients together until smooth, blending the ice cubes last. Drink immediately or refrigerate for a day.

Serves 1–2.

Note: You may use regular dairy yogurt instead of the Almond Yogurt Drink if you prefer.

MINTY CAROB SMOOTHIE

» 4–6 dates (honey or medjool), pitted
» 2 cups Pumpkin Seed Milk or other milk (chapter 5)
» 2 bananas, fresh or frozen
» 2 Tbsp. carob powder (or cacao powder)
» 1 Tbsp. maca powder
» ½ tsp. mineral greens
» 8–10 mint leaves or 3–5 drops peppermint oil
» 1 pinch sea salt (optional)
» 2 cups ice cubes (optional)

Soak the dates in the Pumpkin Seed Milk for 15 minutes to soften them. (If the dates are not hard or if you have a commercial blender, you can skip this step.) Blend all ingredients together until smooth, blending the ice cubes last. To add the peppermint oil extract, dip a clean toothpick in the oil and add one drop from the toothpick. For a

Detox Delish

stronger mint flavor, repeat the step with a clean toothpick. Drink immediately or store in the refrigerator for a day.

Serves 1–2.

Note: Try replacing the mint oil with a few fresh peppermint leaves. Feel free to use another milk.

No-Egg Nog

- » 1½ cups Almond Cream (chapter 5)
- » 6–8 dates (honey or medjool), pitted and de-crowned
- » ¼ cup cashews
- » 1 Tbsp. maca powder
- » ½ tsp. vanilla extract
- » ¼ tsp. nutmeg
- » ⅛ tsp. turmeric
- » 3–5 drops stevia
- » Pinch sea salt (optional)
- » 2 cups ice cubes (optional)

Soak cashews in water for two hours. Then drain and rinse them. Blend all ingredients together until smooth. Drink immediately or store in the refrigerator for a day.

Serves 1–2.

Pumpkin Pie Malt

- » 1½ cups cubed pumpkin or sweet potato
- » 2 bananas, fresh or frozen
- » 1 cup rejuvelac, coconut water, or water
- » 2 Tbsp. honey or liquid sweetener (or 4–6 drops stevia)
- » 1 Tbsp. maca powder (optional)
- » ½ tsp. vanilla extract
- » ⅛ tsp. cinnamon
- » ⅛ tsp. allspice
- » Pinch sea salt (optional)
- » 2 cups ice cubes (optional)

Blend the ingredients together until smooth, blending the ice cubes last. Drink immediately or refrigerate for a day.

Serves 1–2.

108

STRAWBERRY AND BLACK SESAME

» 2 Tbsp. black sesame seeds
» 2 cups strawberries, fresh or frozen
» 2 bananas, fresh or frozen
» 1 cup water
» 2 Tbsp. honey or liquid sweetener (or 4–6 drops stevia)
» 2 cups ice (optional)

Soak black sesame seeds in water for two hours, and then drain and rinse. Blend sesame seeds, strawberries, bananas, water, honey, and ice together until smooth. Drink immediately or store in the refrigerator for a day.

Serves 1–2.

Note: Soaking the sesame seeds makes them easier to digest and absorb nutrients, but sometimes I'll just throw them in without soaking or soak them over night when I'm in a hurry in the morning.

Health note: Black sesame seeds are an Asian remedy for reversing gray hair. They are a rich source of calcium.

GREEN STRENGTH IN A SHAKE

» 2 cups chopped kale, packed (or 2 handfuls kale)
» 2 cups water
» 1 medium avocado
» 3 Tbsp. honey or liquid sweetener (or 4–6 drops stevia)
» 1 Tbsp. cacao or carob powder
» 2 Tbsp. nut/seed butter
» ½ tsp. mineral greens (spirulina, chlorella, etc.)
» 2 bananas
» 2 cups ice cubes (optional)

Blend all ingredients together until smooth, blending the ice cubes last. Drink immediately or refrigerate for a day.

Serves 1–2.

Note: This power-packed energy drink is a liquid meal for people on the go.

BLENDED BROTHS AND SOUPS

Garnishes can be left out if doing a liquid or blended detox.

BUTTERNUT SQUASH

This soup is truly a comfort food.

» ¼ cup cashews
» 2 cups Almond Milk or other milk (chapter 5)
» 3 cups pumpkin or butternut squash, peeled and cubed
» ½ tsp. onion powder
» ¼ tsp. cumin
» ¼ tsp. sea salt
» Dash cayenne pepper

Garnish

» Cashew Sour Cream (chapter 5)
» Pinch minced parsley
» Pinch cayenne pepper

Soak the cashews in water for two hours, then drain and rinse. Blend the cashews and Almond Milk until smooth. Add the pumpkin or butternut squash, onion powder, cumin, sea salt, and cayenne pepper and blend again until smooth. Garnish with Cashew Sour Cream, minced parsley, and a pinch of cayenne pepper. Serve fresh or heated. Store in the refrigerator in an airtight container for up to two days.

Serves 2–4.

Note: Another milk can be replaced for the Pumpkin Seed Milk.

CHILLED HONEYDEW

» 4 cups honeydew melon, cut into 1-inch pieces, frozen
» 2 cups Almond Milk (chapter 5)
» ¼ cup lime juice
» 1 Tbsp. chopped mint leaves
» ¼ tsp. sea salt (optional or to taste)
» 1 cup ice cubes

Garnish (optional)

- » Mint sprigs
- » Cashew Sour Cream (chapter 5)
- » Drizzled honey or liquid sweetener

Blend all the ingredients except the garnishes until smooth. Serve immediately while chilled, adding garnishes as desired.

Serves 2–4.

CLEANSING MISO BROTH

- » 4 cups water
- » 3 Tbsp. miso
- » 1 Tbsp. grated ginger root
- » Dash cayenne pepper
- » Pinch dulse
- » Pinch sea salt (optional or to taste)

In a glass jar with a lid, combine ingredients and shake well (or blend in order to dissolve the miso thoroughly). Serve fresh or heated.

Serves 2–4.

Note: If you are avoiding soy products, buy a miso made from chickpeas or barley. I often drink this savory broth in between juice and smoothie detoxes.

CORN CHOWDER

- » ½ cup cashews
- » 1 cup water
- » 3¼ cups sweet corn kernels
- » 1 tsp. honey or liquid sweetener
- » ¼ tsp. black pepper
- » ¼ tsp. sea salt

Soak the cashews in water for two hours, then drain and rinse. Set aside 3 cups kernels in a medium bowl. Blend the cashews and water until smooth. Add in the remaining ¼ cup kernels, honey, black pepper, and salt until smooth. Pour the blended mixture into the bowl of 3 cups of kernels and gently fold in. Serve immediately or refrigerate in an airtight container for up to two days.

Serves 4–6.

Detox Delish

CREAMY BROCCOFLOWER

- » ¼ cup cashews
- » 2 cups Almond Milk (chapter 5)
- » 3 cups chopped broccoflower
- » 1 Tbsp. white sesame seeds
- » 2 Tbsp. liquid aminos or natural soy sauce
- » 2 Tbsp. chopped parsley
- » 1-inch chunk onion
- » ¼ tsp. black pepper
- » ¼ tsp. garlic powder
- » Pinch sea salt (optional)

Garnish

- » Pinch minced parsley
- » Pinch black pepper

Soak the cashews for two hours, then drain and rinse. Blend the cashews and Almond Milk until smooth. Add the remaining ingredients and blend again until smooth. Serve fresh or heated, garnished with minced parsley and black pepper. Store in the refrigerator in an airtight container for up to two days.

Serves 2–4.

Note: You can easily replace the broccoflower with half broccoli and half cauliflower in this recipe.

CREAMY CASHEW MUSHROOM

- » ½ cup cashews
- » 2 cups rejuvelac, water, or coconut water
- » 2 cups chopped mushrooms (button, cremini, shiitake, etc.)
- » 1 Tbsp. liquid aminos or natural soy sauce
- » 1 Tbsp. miso
- » 1 thin slice garlic
- » ¼ tsp. sesame oil
- » Pinch white pepper
- » Pinch sea salt

Garnish

- » Mushroom slices
- » Pinch black pepper

» 1 Tbsp. minced parsley

Soak the cashews in water for two hours, then drain and rinse. Blend the cashews and rejuvelac, water, or coconut water until smooth. Add the mushrooms, liquid aminos or soy sauce, miso, garlic, sesame oil, white pepper, and sea salt. Blend again until smooth. Garnish with mushroom slices, black pepper, and minced parsley. Serve fresh or heated. Store in the refrigerator in an airtight container for up to two days.

Serves 2–4.

Note: Try a button, cremini, or, for a Japanese twist, a shiitake mushroom. For a different texture, you can blend half of the mushrooms until smooth and pulse the others in so it is slightly chunky.

CURRIED COCONUT-MANGO

» 3 cups mango cubes or slices, fresh or frozen
» 1¼ cups Almond Milk (chapter 5)
» 1¼ cups coconut water
» ½ cup orange juice
» 1 Tbsp. coconut oil
» ½ tsp. curry powder or cumin
» 1 or 2 pinches cayenne
» 1 pinch sea salt (optional or to taste)

Garnish

» Cashew Sour Cream (chapter 5)
» Drizzled honey or liquid sweetener
» Pinch cayenne pepper

Blend all the ingredients until smooth. Serve immediately, garnished with Cashew Sour Cream, honey, and cayenne pepper, or store in the refrigerator in an airtight container for up to two days.

Serves 2–4.

Note: I prefer using frozen mango and adding a cup of ice to chill this soup. This is a refreshingly cool delight on a warm day.

PEPPERED CELERY BISQUE

- » 3 cups chopped celery
- » 2 cups Almond Milk (chapter 5)
- » ¼ cup cashews
- » 2 Tbsp. miso
- » 1 Tbsp. chopped parsley
- » 2 Tbsp. diced onion
- » ¼ tsp. green mineral powder (spirunina, chlorella, etc.)
- » ⅛ tsp. black pepper
- » ⅛ tsp. garlic powder
- » Pinch white pepper
- » Pinch sea salt (optional or to taste)

Garnish

- » Pinch black pepper

Soak the cashews for two hours and then drain and rinse. Blend the cashews and Almond Milk until smooth. Add the remaining ingredients and blend again until smooth. Serve immediately, garnished with black pepper, or store in the refrigerator in an airtight container for up to two days.

Serves 2–4.

Note: Celery is a natural source of sodium, so this may be savory enough for your taste buds without the extra salt.

SPICY TOMATO BROTH

- » 4 large tomatoes
- » 1 large cucumber
- » 2 Tbsp. miso
- » Dash white pepper
- » Dash cayenne
- » Dash chipotle
- » Pinch sea salt (optional or to taste)

Juice the tomatoes and cucumber. In a glass jar with a lid, combine juice and all other ingredients and shake well or blend in order to dissolve the miso thoroughly. Serve fresh or heated.

Serves 2–4.

CHAPTER 8

Salad Basics: No More Boring Salads!

*I*F YOUR RESTAURANT experience starts off great, with you ordering a salad, but then ends up lousy, with you ordering off the dessert menu because you didn't feel satisfied, don't feel discouraged. The salad was simply unsatisfactory in terms of nutrient-density and flavor balance. What is more boring than a garden salad? Perhaps its cousin, the chef salad. And then there are those dressings. Even a good salad can be ruined by the toxic-laden concoctions often disguised as dressings.

I admit I have discreetly brought little packets of nuts and seeds or small bottles of flaxseed or olive oil in my purse to restaurants to add to my salads. This really goes against the grain of social etiquette, and I haven't done this for a while now since dining out is more about the people and good conversations. The point is that when a salad is prepared well, it can make a complete meal. Whether you add your choice of meats, tofu, or eggs is totally up to you.

BUILDING BLOCKS OF A GOOD SALAD

Here are a few guidelines of building a satisfaction-guaranteed, plant-based salad. There are many more options for your salad, but the beauty of the list below is these are items you do not have to prepare ahead of time; chances are they are already in your refrigerator or pantry!

Choose a base
Common salad bases are cabbage, kale, Romaine, spinach, arugula, and butter lettuce. Can you think of another leafy green? Great! Nearly any produce can be the star player in a salad, from leafy greens to cauliflower.

Choose fresh toppings

This is your chance to clear out the refrigerator or browse the produce aisle for some new items to top your salad. Some of my favorite salad toppings include but are not limited to shredded beets and carrots, cubed avocado, diced celery, cubed apples and pears, sprouts (alfalfa, broccoli, etc.), and supremed grapefruit and oranges.

Supreming Citrus

To supreme citrus, take a paring knife and cut off the top and bottom. Rest the fruit on one flattened side. Cut away the peel, leaving no pith. Between each membrane, cut out the citrus sections.

Squeeze, drizzle, sprinkle

Salad dressings don't have to take a lot of work. In fact, they don't even need a recipe. Your dressing could be as simple as squeezing half a lemon onto your salad or splashing on a spoonful of apple cider vinegar. However, chances are you have one ingredient of each category listed below in your kitchen, so experiment. Choose at least one item from each category below and think in terms of spoonful sizes.

1. Fat: Drizzle olive oil, flaxseed oil, or sesame oil over your salad.

2. Sour: Squeeze half an orange, lemon, or lime, or splash in some apple cider vinegar.

3. Sweet: Drizzle on a bit of honey or liquid sweetener.

4. Savory: Drizzle on some natural soy sauce or sprinkle on some sea salt.

Add small amounts of big flavor

Choose some fresh minced herbs, such as basil, cilantro, mint, or parsley. Zest an orange, lemon, or lime. A little bit of seaweed sprinkled on my salad is a savory treat. Add two big spoonfuls of a fermented vegetable, such as my Low-Salt Kimchee (chapter 9), Red Cabbage Kraut (chapter 5) or the cubed beets left over from the Ruby Red Kvass (chapter 10). These savory cultured foods not only help in the digestion by adding probiotics and extra nutrition, but they also provide the X factor of flavor.

Add crunch

Salads often lack the texture of crunch. If I make enough salad for more than one day, I'll leave these foods out, adding them in right before eating to prevent sogginess. I'll often choose one or two of the following to make my salad more energy-packed with the added crunchy texture: pumpkin seeds, sunflower seeds, sesame seeds, ground flaxseed, almonds, walnuts, cashews, and macadamia nuts.

SALAD RECIPES

MASSAGED KALE

- » 2 bunches kale (at least 1 lb.)
- » ½ tsp. sea salt (optional or to taste)
- » 2 lemons, squeezed
- » 2 Tbsp. olive oil
- » 2 Tbsp. flaxseed oil

After de-stemming the kale, chiffonade the kale by tightly rolling the leaves up. Then thinly slice the rolls.

Add the salt and lemon juice and leave five minutes so the salt and citrus break down the kale. Massage the kale about five minutes or until tender. Add in the remaining ingredients. Store in an airtight container in the refrigerator for up to three days.

Makes 2 meals or 4 servings (as side dishes).

Note: Massaged kale makes a complete lunch, but I often add a cooked side along with salads, especially in the cold months. If I'm doing a detox, I'll just do the salad. I love it when people try this salad because most often they can't believe kale, which is wiry unless boiled, steamed, or fried, can taste so tender and good.

ASIAN CABBAGE SALAD

- » 1 head white cabbage (2–3 lb.)
- » ½–¾ tsp. sea salt (optional or to taste)
- » 2 Tbsp. lemon juice
- » 1 orange or grapefruit, supremed
- » 1 cup chopped parsley
- » 2 Tbsp. orange or grapefruit juice (from leftover pulp)
- » 2 Tbsp. apple cider vinegar
- » 2 Tbsp. white sesame seeds
- » 1 Tbsp. olive oil or flaxseed oil
- » 1 Tbsp. honey
- » 1 tsp. sesame oil
- » ½ cup almonds, chopped

In a food processor or by hand, thinly slice the cabbage. In a big bowl, add the cabbage with the salt and lemon juice and toss so the contents are coated. Massage it for about one minute to tenderize the cabbage. Supreme the orange or grapefruit and set aside. Squeeze juice from the leftover pulp in with the cabbage. Toss in remaining ingredients, adding the almonds right before serving to preserve their crunchiness. Store in an airtight container in the refrigerator up to three days.

Makes 2 meals or 4 servings.

BAKED CRUSTED SALMON (COOKED OPTION)

- » 10–12 oz. salmon
- » 1 egg
- » 1 Tbsp. miso

Cut the salmon into 1-inch chunks. Using a whisk or fork, combine the egg and miso until smooth. Mix the salmon in with the egg-miso batter.

Note: Tofu can be used instead of salmon for a vegetarian option. When buying tofu, look for non-GMO, organic brands. You can replace the egg with 2 tsp. chia seeds ground in a coffee grinder and mixed with 3 Tbsp. water.

Coating

- » ½ cup macadamia nuts
- » ½ cup almonds
- » ½ tsp. sea salt
- » 1 clove garlic

In a small, dry food processor, grind the macadamia nuts, almonds, garlic (peeled), and salt until a crumbly texture is reached. Pulsing the ingredients in a dry blender works as well.

Then coat the salmon in the nut mixture. Bake the salmon at 350 degrees Fahrenheit for 15 minutes or until it is flaky. (If you are using tofu rather than salmon, it can also be baked at 350 degrees Fahrenheit for 15 minutes.) Add as an optional topping to Asian Cabbage Salad, and store extra in an airtight container up to three days.

CRAN-APPLE WALNUT SALAD WITH CASHEW CHEESE

- » 1–2 bunches romaine lettuce, chopped (1 lb. romaine)
- » 2 Tbsp. apple cider vinegar
- » 3 Tbsp. olive oil
- » ¼ tsp. sea salt
- » 2 Tbsp. honey or liquid sweetener
- » ¼ tsp. black pepper
- » 1 cup chopped walnuts
- » 1 cup chopped apples
- » ¾ cup cranberries
- » ½ cup Cashew Cheese (chapter 5)

Mix the vinegar, oil, salt, liquid sweetener, and pepper in with the lettuce. Before serving, top the salad with the walnuts, apples, cranberries, and cheese. (Break the cheese up into bite size pieces.) Store in an airtight container in the refrigerator for up to three days.

Makes 2 meals or 4 servings.

Note: Cranberries are often sweetened with sugar. At the local organic co-op I found cranberries in the bulk section sweetened with apple juice. You can also replace the cranberries with raisins or goji berries. Store them in an airtight container in a cool, dry place.

HORSERADISH COLLARD SLAW

Slaw

» 2 bunches collard greens
» ¼ tsp. sea salt
» 1 lemon, squeezed

After de-stemming the greens, tightly roll up the collard greens and slice them into fine shreds. Add the salt and lemon juice and leave five to ten minutes so the salt and citrus break down the greens. Then massage the greens until they are tender (Or, if you are in a hurry, you can start massaging them right away).

Note: Kale works in place of the collard greens.

Dressing

» ½ cup cashews
» ¼ cup water
» 1 Tbsp. grated horseradish
» 2 Tbsp. olive oil
» 1 Tbsp. miso
» 1 tsp. wasabi powder or paste
» 1 tsp. onion powder
» ½ tsp. garlic powder
» ½ tsp. black pepper
» ¼ tsp. sea salt (or to taste)

For the dressing, whirl all the ingredients together in a blender.

Garnish

» ½ cup sunflower seeds

Before serving, combine the collard greens and dressing and top with the sunflower seeds. Store in an airtight container in the refrigerator up to three days. For remaining salad dressing, store in an airtight container in the refrigerator up to one week.

Makes 2 meals or 4 servings (as side dishes).

ICEBERG WEDGES WITH PEPPERCORN RANCH AND NUTTY PARMESAN

Salad

» 2 heads iceberg lettuce

Cut each head of iceberg in half and then cut each half into thirds, making 6 wedges per head. Makes 12 wedges. You can also just chop this up for one huge salad.

Dressing

» 1 cup cashews, soaked two hours, drained, and rinsed
» 1½ cups rejuvelac or water
» 2 Tbsp. lemon juice
» 2 Tbsp. olive oil or flaxseed oil
» 2 Tbsp. miso
» 1 tsp. crush black peppercorns
» ½ tsp. onion powder
» ¼ tsp. garlic powder
» ½ tsp. sea salt (optional or to taste)

For the dressing, blend all the ingredients until smooth.

Parmesan

» ¼ cup flaxseed
» ¼ cup nutritional yeast
» 1 cup macadamia nuts
» 1 cup almonds
» 3 cloves garlic
» 1½ tsp. sea salt (optional or to taste)

To make the parmesan, grind the flaxseed to form a flour consistency in a dry blender, and then add it to a bowl along with the nutritional yeast. Pulse the remaining ingredients in the blender one cup at a time until a crumbly texture is formed. Stop the blender to loosen the mixture with a rubber spatula as needed. Mix nut mixture in bowl with the flaxseed and yeast. Serve immediately or refrigerate in an airtight container for up to two weeks. (This recipe makes over 2 cups of parmesan.)

Note: I used the light-colored, golden flaxseed for this recipe so the parmesan has a white appearance similar to traditional parmesan. However, any shade, brown or golden, of flaxseed will work for this recipe.

Before serving, add a couple dollops of dressing over each wedge and garnish with a spoonful of the nutty parmesan. Serve immediately or store the dressing in an airtight container in the refrigerator up to one week. The parmesan can be stored in an airtight container in the refrigerator up to two weeks.

Makes 2 meals or 4 servings.

Note: Despite it's bad rap for not ranking nutritionally compared to kale or collard greens, I love iceberg lettuce. It offers a wonderful crunch and offers a high-water content. Adding arugula or a spring mix to iceberg adds variety and more nutrients if desired.

KALE SEAWEED SALAD

- » 2 bunches kale (at least 1 lb.)
- » ½ tsp. sea salt (optional or to taste)
- » 3 Tbsp. apple cider vinegar
- » ¾ cup dried arame seaweed (15 oz.)
- » ¼ cup sesame seeds
- » 3 Tbsp. tamari or natural soy sauce
- » 1 Tbsp. grated ginger
- » 1 Tbsp. olive oil
- » 1 Tbsp. flaxseed oil
- » 1 tsp. sesame oil

After de-stemming the kale, chiffonade the kale by tightly rolling the leaves up and then thinly slicing the rolls. Add the salt and vinegar and leave it for five minutes so the salt and vinegar break down the kale. Massage the kale for about five minutes or until tender. Soak the seaweed for twenty minutes and then drain. Add in the remaining ingredients with the kale. Store in an airtight container in the refrigerator for up to three days.

Makes 2 meals or 4 servings.

QUINOA-SHIITAKE RICE (COOKED OPTION)

- » 1 cup rice
- » ½ cup quinoa

- » 1½ cups water
- » ¾ cup sliced shiitake (or favorite mushroom)
- » ⅓ cup raisins or diced dates
- » 2 Tbsp. natural soy sauce (tamari, Bragg liquid aminos, etc.)
- » ¼ tsp. minced or grated ginger
- » ¼ tsp. sesame oil
- » Pinch sea salt

Garnish

- » ½ tsp. sesame seeds

Soak the rice and quinoa, separately or together, for eight hours, and then drain and rinse until the water is no longer cloudy. Bring the quinoa, rice, and water to boil. As soon as the boiling point is reached, turn the burner to low and cover it with a lid. Simmer 12 to 15 minutes. Turn heat off and gently fold in the remaining ingredients, fluffing the contents as you go. Lid and let sit ten minutes. Garnish with sesame seeds.

Serves 4.

Note: Bringing the boil down to a simmer allows less water to be used and helps prevent rice from sticking to the bottom of the pan.

LIGHTLY SEASONED BRUSSELS SPROUTS WITH AVOCADO VINAIGRETTE

Brussels sprouts

- » 1 lb. brussels sprouts, shredded
- » ½ lb. red radishes (or one bunch), shredded
- » 1 Tbsp. apple cider vinegar
- » 1 Tbsp. olive oil
- » 1 Tbsp. dulse flakes
- » ½ tsp. sea salt

To make the salad, toss everything together.

Dressing

- » 1 cup cubed avocado (about 1 medium avocado)
- » ½ cup rejuvelac, water, or milk
- » ¼ cup lime juice

- » 2 Tbsp. olive oil
- » 2 Tbsp. apple cider vinegar
- » 1 Tbsp. miso
- » ¼ cup chopped jalapeño
- » ½ tsp. sea salt
- ⁕ ⅓ cup sunflower seeds (garnish)

To make the dressing, blend ingredients (except the garnish) together until smooth. The salad and the dressing are served separately with the dressing and sunflower seeds added by each person. The salad and dressing can be stored in airtight containers in the refrigerator up to three days.

Serves 4–6.

Two Flowers Pilaf

- » 2 heads cauliflower (about 2 lb.), diced
- » ¼ cup lemon juice
- » ½ tsp. sea salt
- » ¾ cup sunflower seeds
- » ¾ cup finely diced celery
- » ½ cup nutritional yeast (optional)
- » ½ cup minced onions
- » 2 Tbsp. olive oil
- » 2 Tbsp. flaxseed oil
- » 1 tsp. lemon zest (or zest one lemon)

Chop up the cauliflower into popcorn size. You can also pulse larger chunks of cauliflower in a food processor. Place the cauliflower, lemon juice, and salt in a large bowl. Massage for about five minutes or until the cauliflower becomes tender. Fold in the remaining ingredients. Serve immediately or refrigerate in an airtight container for up to three days.

Makes 2 meals or 4 servings.

Note: A medley of cauliflower, sunflower seeds, and citrus juices make this one of my favorites. This salad tastes even better the next day once all the flavors combine nicely with the cauliflower.

CHAPTER 9

Raw Cuisine Around the World

YOU JUST FINISHED a detox and now feel the cleanest and most energized you've felt in years. Soon after, you quickly return to the SAD, your sad state of normal. Is there life after a cleanse? Remember detoxes and fasts are not diets in disguise. Diets only promise short-term results. Just as you entered into your detox and fast for renewal and cleansing, you must exit the detox and fast with the same perspective by transitioning into a new lifestyle of cleaner eating. We are not searching for perfection here, but a real lifestyle change. For some it may be a goal of adding one smoothie or juice a day. For others it may be making sure each meal is half vegetables, either raw or cooked. For others, it may be adding something raw to each meal.

One of the best ways to transition out of a juice and smoothie fast is to start introducing raw foods, prepared or eaten whole, into the diet. Salads and smoothies are my go-to meals. However, I enjoy preparing raw-food cuisine as celebration foods to share with friends and show them just how delicious raw food can be. This section provides a creative menu to show you how raw food can be so much more than salads alone. Celebrate creation's abundant and delicious supply of fruits, vegetables, nuts, and seeds with me.

Each menu consists of an appetizer, side dish, main dish, and dessert. Some of the main dishes are as simple as throwing together a salad. For some of the main dishes that take more time or have special ingredients, there will be a salad conversion option, using the main ingredients of the main dish and tossing it with some green leafy vegetables for a refreshingly light and flavorful salad!

MAKE RAW NOT WAR (AMERICAN)

This menu is the closest to home. I've often heard that everything tastes better with bacon and butter. I was raised on a vegetable farm, but I also raised steer for work projects. I'm also thankful for my childhood drinking organic and unpasteurized milk from the neighbor's cows and goats. Since my younger years I've transitioned more to a plant-based lifestyle, but I am not a strict vegan or vegetarian. Make Raw Not War is a celebration of traditional favorites turned into plant-based gems, not complete without my Beet Bacon and plant-based butter.

Appetizer

OPEN-FACED EGGLESS SALAD ON DILL BREAD

- » Dill Bread (see recipe)
- » 1 head butter leaf lettuce
- » Eggless Salad (see recipe)
- » Dill sprig
- » Dill Pickle Slice (see recipe, optional)

Dill Bread

- » 1 cup zucchini peels and parts (leftover from the Mac and Cheese With Beet Bacon main dish recipe)
- » 1 cup walnuts
- » 2 Tbsp. olive oil
- » 2 Tbsp. honey or liquid sweetener
- » ½ cup ground flaxseed (also called flaxseed meal)
- » ½ cup almond flour or leftover nut or seed pulp
- » 2 Tbsp. nutritional yeast
- » 2 tsp. psyllium husk
- » 2 Tbsp. dried dill, crushed + ½ tsp. for topping
- » ¼ tsp. salt
- » 9 butter lettuce leaves (garnish)

In a food processor fitted with an S-blade, combine the zucchini, walnuts, olive oil, and honey until a crumbled texture is formed. (It is OK if the zucchini is a little clumpy at this point.) In a bowl add this mixture and fold in the flaxseed, almond flour, nutritional yeast, psyllium husk, and dried dill. Leave salt aside.

Spread out onto one nonstick drying sheet or parchment paper sheet into a square about ¼-inch thick. Score two ways horizontal and two ways vertical, making nine pieces. If using a round food dehydrator with a hole in the middle for ventilation, simply shape the bread mixture in the circular trays and score them as desire with a butter knife or spatula. Sprinkle the salt over the top of the mixture.

Dehydrate at 115 degrees Fahrenheit for three hours. Flip onto a screen tray. Dehydrate twelve to eighteen hours. Place a butter lettuce leaf on each piece of bread.

Makes 9 slices.

Dill Pickles

» 2 cups sliced cucumbers
» 1½ cups water
» ½ cup apple cider vinegar
» 6–10 sprigs dill
» 2 cloves garlic, minced
» 1 tsp. sea salt

Place the cucumber slices in a jar with all of the other ingredients. Let stand at least one hour or overnight on the countertop before serving. These pickles will keep in the refrigerator for up to one month.

Makes 2 cups.

Note: Use a cheese cutter to slice the cucumber with ridges.

Eggless Salad

» ¾ cup young Thai coconut meat (1–2 coconuts)
» 1 cup Cashew Sour Cream or dairy sour cream (chapter 5)
» ⅓ cup finely diced celery
» ¼ cup diced dill pickles
» 1 Tbsp. miso
» 1 Tbsp. nutritional yeast (optional)
» 1 tsp. lemon juice
» 1 tsp. white chia seeds
» ½ tsp. mustard powder
» ¼ tsp. turmeric

- » ¼ tsp. sea salt
- » Pinch white pepper

Garnish

- » Dill sprig
- » Dill pickle slice (optional)
- » 1 tsp. dill

Cut the coconut meat into thin slices and then chop into about ¾-inch long pieces. Place in a colander lined with a paper towel to soak up excess water. Use a paper towel to squeeze out excess juice from the pickles and celery if wet. Fold in the remaining ingredients with the young coconut meat.

Chill one hour.

Makes about 2 cups.

To assemble the Open-Faced Eggless Salad on Dill Bread, layer each slice of bread (with a butter lettuce leaf already on top) with a scoop of Eggless Salad and garnish with a dill sprig or dill pickles and dill.

Young Thai Coconut Meat

Young coconuts, often referred to as young Thai coconuts, have tender flesh and are full of refreshing coconut water. They have a diamond-shaped crown opposed to the round coconuts often sold with a firmer, dryer flesh. An alternative to harvesting the coconut meat by hand is to buy the coconut meat frozen and sliced into strips, often found at Asian food markets or natural food stores.

To get young Thai coconut meat, use a butcher's knife, or heavy knife, to cut off the crown-shaped point of the coconut. Punch a hole in the exposed shell to pry off the circular top. After draining out and enjoying the coconut water, scoop out the coconut meat. In its tender state, it should scoop out with a spoon or rubber spatula. Before using the flesh, use a paring knife to shave off the little wooden pieces still attached to the coconut meat.

Side dish

PEAS AND CARROTS WITH BUTTER

Vegetables

» 2 cups peas
» 1 cup diced carrots
» 1 tsp. olive oil
» Pinch sea salt
» Pinch black pepper

Combine ingredients together. For a warmed option, place on a shallow baking sheet or no-stick drying sheet on parchment paper and dehydrate for one or two hours at 115 degrees Fahrenheit.

Serves 4.

Butter

» ⅓ cup cashews
» ½ cup water
» ½ cup coconut oil
» 2 Tbsp. lecithin
» 1 Tbsp. miso
» 1 Tbsp. apple cider vinegar
» 1 Tbsp. olive oil
» ¼ tsp. sea salt
» ⅛ tsp. turmeric

Soak the cashews for two hours, then drain and rinse them. Blend all the ingredients until creamy smooth. Pour into a square container and chill for four hours in the refrigerator or one hour in the freezer. Store in an airtight container in the refrigerator up to two weeks.

Makes 1½ cups.

To serve the peas with butter, add a small dollop of butter to each serving or a big dollop if the vegetables are served in a bowl.

Lecithin

You can swap either soy or sunflower lecithin depending on your preferences.

Main dish

MAC AND CHEESE WITH BEET BACON

Noodles

» 4 medium zucchini

To make the noodles, use a spiralizer or vegetable peeler.

Cheese sauce

» 1 cup Cashew Sour Cream or dairy sour cream (chapter 5)
» ½ cup minced cauliflower
» ¼ cup nutritional yeast (optional)
» ¼ tsp. chipotle powder
» ¼ tsp. turmeric powder
» 1 Tbsp. olive oil
» 1 Tbsp. lemon juice
» 1 Tbsp. finely sliced onions + 1 Tbsp. for garnishing
» ½ tsp. onion powder
» ⅓ tsp. sea salt (or to taste)

To make the cheese sauce, blend all the ingredients together until smooth. Scrape down the sides of the blender with a rubber spatula as needed.

Beet Bacon

» 5 to 6 Chioggia beetroots (about 1 lb.)
» 2½ tsp. sea salt
» 2 Tbsp. olive oil
» 2 Tbsp. natural soy sauce (tamari or Bragg liquid amino acids)
» 2 Tbsp. maple syrup
» 2 Tbsp. apple cider vinegar (or Flame Detox in chapter 10)
» 1 tsp. black pepper
» ½ tsp. chipotle powder
» ¾ cup ground flaxseed

Using a mandoline, thinly slice the beetroots. Mix the beetroots with all ingredients except for the ground flaxseed. Transfer beet mixture to a pan. Let marinate for four hours or overnight in the refrigerator. Turn beets over so all areas are marinated. Sprinkle the flaxseed over the beets and toss. Let sit twenty to thirty minutes so the flaxseed soaks up the marinated juices. Place beets single layered on four dehydrator screen trays. Dehydrate at 115 degrees Fahrenheit for six hours. Flip beet bacon over. Dehydrate for another twelve hours or until crispy.

Note: Red beetroots work well with this recipe. The Chioggia beets have a red and white rainbow scheme that resembles bacon, so I used these. Beet bacon is good and salty and works well in soups, on salads, and even in sandwiches. However, if you eat it alone as a chip, cut the salt amount in half to 1¼ tsp.

To serve Mac and Cheese With Beet Bacon, combine the cheese sauce with the noodles until all the noodles are coated. For any leftover cheese sauce, store in an airtight container up to five days, separate from the noodles. Toss with the beet bacon.

Serves 4.

Dessert

FUDGE B-RAW-NIE WITH WALNUTS

- » ½ cup cashews
- » ½ cup maple syrup
- » ¾ cup cacao butter, liquefied
- » ¼ cup coconut oil, liquefied
- » 1 cup cacao powder or carob powder
- » ⅛ tsp. sea salt
- » 4–6 drops stevia
- » 1 tsp. vanilla extract
- » 1½ cup almond flour (or leftover nut or seed pulp)
- » ½ cup chopped walnuts

Soak cashews for two hours, and then drain and rinse. Blend cashews, maple syrup, cacao butter, and coconut oil until smooth. Blend in the cacao powder, salt, stevia, and vanilla extract until combined. Scrape down the sides of the blender with a rubber spatula as needed. Pour the fudge batter into a bowl and then fold in the almond flour. Pour the mixture into an 8 x 8 pan lined with parchment paper. Top with walnuts and press them down part way. Chill in the refrigerator for two hours or in the freezer for thirty minutes. Store in an airtight container in the refrigerator up to two weeks. Makes one 8 x 8 inch rectangle.

GREAT RAW OF CHINA (CHINESE)

From eating the spicy flavors of Sichuan to the savory and the sweet dishes of Jiangsu, living in China taught me to appreciate how vast and unique one country's cuisine can be. From the spice markets to China's growing organic farms, China has so much to offer in terms of ethnic flavors, herbs, and spices. It was in Beijing where I started teaching raw-food classes, featuring one of Beijing's signature dishes, zha jiang noodles, a traditional favorite of wheat noodles with pork topping and fresh vegetables. Great Raw of China celebrates a fresh veggie outlook on this traditional favorite.

Appetizer

PAI HUANG GUA

» 3 medium cucumbers (about 1 lb.)
» 2 Tbsp. apple cider vinegar
» 1 tsp. sesame oil
» 3 cloves garlic, crushed
» ¼ tsp. sea salt (optional and to taste)
» ⅛ tsp. cayenne pepper (or red pepper flakes)

Slice the cucumbers longways in half, then slice diagonally into half-inch cubes. With the side of your knife, smash the cucumbers. Combine all the ingredients together and serve. Refrigerator in an airtight container for up to five days.

Serves 4 to 6 (meant to eat in small amounts).

Note: This Chinese cold dish, meaning "smashed cucumbers," is traditionally made with white vinegar. The crushed cucumbers soak up the flavors, so this dish is even better the next day.

Side dish

CABBAGE OYSTER SHELLS WITH HONEY-GINGER PEARLS

Shells

» 8–10 red cabbage leaves

With kitchen scissors shape the cabbage leaves into small rounds and set aside.

Salad

» 2 cups diced pears
» 1 cup cherry tomato halves
» 1 cup diced cucumbers
» ½ cup diced celery
» ½ cup sweet corn kernels

Add the salad contents to a bowl and mix.

Glaze

» 2 Tbsp. honey or agave nectar
» 2 tsp. grated ginger
» ½ tsp. sea salt
» 1 pinch cayenne

Add all of these ingredients to the salad bowl and fold in.

Garnish

» ¾ cup cashews
» Celery leaves
» Cayenne

Add ½ cup or more of the salad to each cabbage shell. Garnish each salad shell with cashews, celery leaves, and a pinch of cayenne. Serve immediately.

Makes 8–10 shells.

Detox Delish

Main dish

ZHA JIANG NOODLES

Noodles

» 4 medium zucchini

To make the noodles, use a spiralizer or vegetable peeler.

Sauce

» ½ cup sunflower seeds
» 2 Tbsp. water
» 2½ cups chopped mushrooms (button, cremini, shiitake, etc.)
» ¼ cup olive oil
» ¼ cup tamari or Bragg liquid aminos (soy sauces)
» 1 Tbsp. miso
» 1 Tbsp. honey
» 1 tsp. grated orange peel
» 1 tsp. grated ginger
» ½ tsp. sesame oil
» ½ tsp. black pepper
» ½ tsp. minced garlic
» ¼ tsp. sea salt (optional)

For the sauce, soak the sunflower seeds for two to four hours, and then rinse and drain. In a food processor combine the sunflower seeds and water. The texture does not have to be perfectly smooth. Add the mushrooms and blend again. Then add the remaining ingredients, stopping occasionally to scrape down the sides of the food processor.

Toppings and Garnish

» 1 cup diced celery
» 1 cup cucumber, julienne sliced
» 1 cup soy bean sprouts
» Celery leaves

Zha jiang mian is traditionally served in separate bowls, dividing the noodles and toppings. The noodles and sauce can be served both warm and cold. For a warmed dish, place in the dehydrator for one to two hours at 115 degrees.

Serves 6–8.

Note: *Zha jiang mian* means "fried sauce noodles," but this recipe is anything but fried. This fresh version has the same flavor without the fried oils and pork.

Dessert

CHINESE ALMOND COOKIES

- » 1½ cups dry cashews
- » 1 cup almonds, peeled or blanched
- » 1 cup coconut flakes
- » ½ cup maple syrup (or liquid sweetener)
- » ½ tsp. vanilla extract
- » ¼ tsp. sea salt
- » 20–22 almonds, peeled and halved

In a food processor, combine the ingredients except the almond halves until a crumbly texture is reached. (You can also use a blender by pulsing one cup's worth of ingredients at a time to form a flour consistency. Then add the crumbled mixture to a bowl and combine with the sweetener, vanilla extract, and salt until a doughy texture is formed.) Roll the dough into little balls and flatten, topping with an almond. Place the cookies directly onto the dehydrator tray and dehydrate at 115 degrees Fahrenheit for eight hours.

Makes 20–22 cookies.

Note: The almonds do not have to be peeled, but to get a white-colored flour, they can be blanched by placing the almonds in boiling water for 60 seconds. Drain and rinse with cold water and pop off the skins. Another alternative is to soak for thirty-six hours, replacing the water every twelve hours. The skins are now more easily removed by peeling or popping off. The soaked almonds will dry out in the food dehydrator.

FRESH PHI-RAW-SOPHY (GREEK)

Not yet having traveled to Greece, I've enjoyed Greek food from restaurants during my travels. Who doesn't like hummus? Traditionally made from garbanzo beans, my hummus recipe comes with a light green twist and uses pumpkin seeds. My first try at a raw version of baklava, now called Bakla-Raw, was at culinary art school. It was a challenging but delightful surprise.

Appetizer

OLIVE AND SUN-DRIED TOMATO FLATBREAD

» 2 cups chopped zucchini
» 1 cup walnuts
» ¼ cup olive oil
» 2 Tbsp. maple syrup
» ½ cup ground flaxseed
» ½ cup almond flour or leftover nut or seed pulp
» 2 Tbsp. nutritional yeast
» 2 tsp. psyllium husk
» ⅔ cup olives, halved
» ½ cup sun-dried tomatoes, soaked in ¼ cup water
» ¼ tsp. sea salt + ¼ tsp. sea salt for topping
» 1 Tbsp. crushed caraway seed

In a food processor fitted with an S-blade, combine the zucchini, walnuts, olive oil, and maple syrup until a crumbled texture is formed. In a bowl, add this mixture and fold in the flaxseed, almond flour, nutritional yeast, psyllium husk, olives, sun-dried tomatoes, caraway seed, and salt. Leave ¼ tsp. salt aside.

Spread out onto one nonstick drying sheet or parchment paper sheet into a round shape about ¼-inch thick. Score across four times until there are eight slices. Sprinkle the remaining salt over the top of the mixture.

Dehydrate at 115 degrees Fahrenheit for three hours. Flip onto a screen tray. Continue dehydrating twelve to eighteen hours.

Note: If using a round food dehydrator with a hole in the middle for ventilation, simply shape the bread mixture in the circular trays and score them as desire with a butter knife or spatula.

Makes 8 slices.

Side dish

PUMPKIN SEED HUMMUS

» 1 cup pumpkin seeds
» ¾ cup cashews
» 1½ cups chopped zucchini
» ½ cup rejuvelac or water
» 3 Tbsp. lemon juice
» 2 Tbsp. miso
» 2 garlic cloves
» ⅓ tsp. sea salt
» 2 Tbsp. olive oil + 1 Tbsp. olive oil for garnish
» ¼ cup nutritional yeast (optional)
» Sprigs of parsley

Soak the pumpkin seeds four to six hours, and then drain and rinse. Soak the cashews two hours, and then drain and rinse. Set aside the nutritional yeast, sprigs of parsley, and 1 Tbsp. olive oil. In a food processor, blend all other ingredients until smooth. Scrape down the sides with a rubber spatula as needed. Stir in the nutritional yeast. Transfer the mixture into a serving bowl and drizzle olive oil over the top and garnish with a sprig or two of parsley. Serve immediately or refrigerate in an airtight container up to three days.

Makes about 4 cups.

Note: Serve this hummus with your favorite crudités, cut veggies, or as a topping for the Olive and Sun-Dried Tomato Flatbread.

Main dish

COLLARD GREEN DOLMAS

Marinade

» ¼ cup olive oil
» 1 Tbsp. lemon juice
» 2 tsp. honey or agave nectar
» 1 tsp. minced garlic
» 1 tsp. sea salt

Blend or mix all the ingredients and add to a shallow bowl or tray.

Wraps

» 12–18 collard green leaves (or any flat leaves)

To prepare the wraps, lay the leaves shiny side down and remove the stems and veins. In a shallow pan coat the leaves with the marinade and then leave them to marinate in the liquid for at least one hour to overnight. This will soften the leaves, making them more pliable to roll.

Filling

» 2 Tbsp. flaxseed
» ½ cup macadamia nuts
» 2 cups minced mushrooms (button, cremini, shiitake, etc.)
» 2 cups minced cauliflower
» ½ cup finely diced dates or raisins
» ½ cup minced onions
» 2 Tbsp. lemon juice
» 2 Tbsp. liquid aminos or natural soy sauce
» 2 Tbsp. minced peppermint
» 1 Tbsp. olive oil
» 1 tsp. black pepper
» ¾ tsp. sea salt
» ¼ tsp. cinnamon
» ¼ tsp. nutmeg

For the filling, in a dry blender pulse the flaxseed into a flour consistency and set aside in a large bowl. Then pulse the macadamia nuts into a crumbly mixture and add to the same bowl. Combine all the ingredients together.

To assemble, place a leaf shiny side down. Add a spoonful or two of the filling, depending on the leaf's size, at the base. Roll the base of the leaf over the mixture and then fold in the sides before rolling the rest of the way.

Makes 12–18 dolmas.

Note: If the dolmas start to unfold, use a toothpick to hold them together and remove before serving. You can also wrap them in plastic wrap for a few hours; this will help the rolls keep their shape after taking the wrap off.

My Big Fat Greek Salad (main dish salad option)

» 1 medium cucumber, cubed
» 1 medium tomato, cubed
» 1 ripe avocado, cubed
» 1 cup olives (any kind)
» 2 Tbsp. apple cider vinegar
» 2 Tbsp. olive oil
» 1 Tbsp. flaxseed oil
» ¼ tsp. black pepper
» 1 garlic, minced
» Pinch sea salt (optional or to taste)
» 1 Tbsp. ground flaxseed
» ½ cup Cashew Cheese (chapter 5)

Toss all ingredients together and enjoy. Top this salad with bite-size Cashew Cheese pieces chunks. Refrigerate in an airtight container up to three days.

Serves 4–6.

Note: This salad is a complete meal that includes multiple good fats, including those ever important omega-3 fatty acids in flaxseed.

Dessert

Bakla-raw

Apple Layers

» 4 apples, large
» 1 lemon, juiced

For the apple phyllo, using a mandoline, slice the apples as thinly as possible. Cut off the rounds to form squares. Coat the apple slices with lemon juice to prevent browning. I also coat my hands in lemon juice when handling and assembling the apple slices. Five slices will be used per serving.

Filling

» 2 cups walnuts
» ⅓ cup maple syrup
» ⅓ cup coconut palm nectar

- » ½ cup dates, pitted and de-crowned
- » 2 tsp. vanilla extract
- » 1 tsp. lemon juice
- » 1 tsp. lemon zest
- » ¾ tsp. cinnamon
- » ¼ tsp. cardamom (optional)
- » ⅛ tsp. mace (optional)
- » ¼ tsp. sea salt

To make the filling, use a food processor to break the walnuts down to the size of grape seeds and set aside. Using a blender, combine the remaining ingredients until smooth. Remove ½ cup of the filling for the topping. Pour remaining mixture into the 4 cups of the walnuts. This topping stores in an airtight container in the refrigerator up to two weeks.

Garnish

- » ½ cup walnuts, chopped
- » ½ cup sauce (taken from filling)
- » ½ tsp. cinnamon

To assemble into one big dessert, layer one apple's worth of slices on bottom layer of an 8 x 8 pan, and then layer on two to three scoops of the filling. Repeat three more times, then garnish with walnuts and more filling, and dust the cinnamon on top.

To assemble individual desserts, start with a square apple slice and then place a spoonful of filling. Repeat using five apple slices per serving. On top of the last apple slice, garnish with the filling, walnuts, and cinnamon.

Makes 8 to 10 individual bakla-raws or one 8 x 8 pan.

Note: The leftover apple remains can be juiced.

FEAST OF RAW-SH HASHANAH (ISRAELI)

Since I was given the opportunity to travel to the Middle East, Israel has been a favorite destination of mine—with everything from the Biblical destinations of the Sea of Galilee to the Upper Room in Jerusalem. Foods in biblical times are still eaten today: dates, raisins and nuts, a variety of cheeses, fresh fruits, and olives.

Also, since my travels, I've not forgotten to fill up on freshly pressed pomegranate juice.

Much of Israeli food consists of fresh salads and dips and sauces, such as hummus and tahini. This meal plan celebrates the ancient ingredients whipped up to remind you of those traditional favorites.

Appetizer

GARLIC AND ONION FLATBREAD

- » 1½ cups chopped zucchini
- » 1 cup walnuts
- » ¼ cup olive oil
- » 2 Tbsp. honey or liquid sweetener
- » 1 clove garlic, minced
- » ½ cup ground flaxseed
- » ½ cup almond flour or leftover nut or seed pulp
- » 2 Tbsp. nutritional yeast
- » 2 tsp. psyllium husk
- » 1 tsp. onion powder
- » ½ tsp. sea salt + ¼ tsp. sea salt for topping
- » ¼ cup thinly sliced onion

In a food processor fitted with an S-blade, combine the zucchini, walnuts, olive oil, honey, and garlic until a crumbled texture is formed. In a bowl, add this mixture and fold in the flaxseed, almond flour, nutritional yeast, psyllium husk, onion powder, sliced onion, and salt. Leave ¼ tsp. salt for the topping.

Spread out onto one nonstick drying sheet or parchment paper sheet into a square about ¼-inch thick. Score two ways horizontally and two ways vertically, making nine pieces. If using a round food dehydrator with a hole in the middle for ventilation, simply shape the bread mixture in the circular trays and score them as you desire with a butter knife or spatula. Sprinkle the salt over the top of the mixture.

Dehydrate at 115 degrees Fahrenheit for three hours. Flip onto a screen tray and continue dehydrate for twelve to eighteen hours.

Makes 9 slices.

Detox Delish

Side dish

CUCUMBER WITH LABENEH

Also spelled "labneh," this is Middle Eastern yogurt-cheese with Lebanese roots. Israelis enjoy labeneh as a breakfast item. Israelis will also dry out the labeneh to form balls and serve with black sesame seeds and olive oil. For Westerners the taste is sort of cream cheese meets yogurt. Either way, it's delicious! It's a wonderful addition to spread on bread or top salads and the main dish, On the Sea of Ga-raw-lee.

» 2 cups Cashew Sour Cream (chapter 5)
» 2 tsp. minced mint
» ½ garlic clove, minced
» Pinch sea salt
» 1 cup diced cucumbers (1 cucumber)

Toppings

» Sprig of mint
» 2 Tbsp. olive oil

Stir together sour cream, mint, garlic, and salt to make the labeneh. Fold in the cucumbers. Garnish with mint and olive oil.

Main dish

ON THE SEA OF GA-RAW-LEE

» 2 large avocados, cubed
» ¾ cup diced tomatoes
» ½ cup sliced olives (any kind)
» ¼ cup minced onion
» 2 tsp. apple cider vinegar
» 1 tsp. honey
» 1 tsp. ground parsley or thyme (fresh or dry)
» 1 tsp. dulse flakes
» Pinch black pepper
» Pinch sea salt

Garnish

» 4 Tbsp. Cucumber With Labeneh (recipe above)
» Parsley or thyme

Slice the avocados in half; the avocado shell will be used to hold the contents. With a spoon scoop out the avocado and cube. In a bowl gently fold all the ingredients except the Cucumbers With Labeneh and parsley sprigs together and scoop into the avocado shells. Spoon 1 Tbsp. Cucumber With Labeneh onto each avocado and top with a parsley sprig. Serve after assembling. Refrigerate in an airtight container for up to one day or the avocados will brown.

Makes 4 servings.

Note: For a variation of the garnish use the labeneh without the cucumber.

IS-RAW-LI SALAD (MAIN DISH SALAD OPTION)

» ¾ cup diced tomatoes
» ½ cup sliced olives (any kind)
» ¼ cup minced onion
» 2 tsp. apple cider vinegar
» 1 tsp. ground thyme (fresh or dry)
» 1 tsp. ground parley (fresh or dry)
» 1 tsp. dulse flakes
» Dash black pepper
» Dash sea salt (optional and to taste)
» 1 bunch spring salad mix (or any kind)
» 1 cucumber, diced
» 1 Tbsp. olive oil
» 1 Tbsp. flaxseed oil
» 4 Tbsp. Cucumber With Labeneh (recipe above)
» Parsley sprigs

Toss all ingredients except the labeneh and parsley together. Top this salad with the same topping as On the Sea of Ga-raw-lee, the Cucumber With Labeneh and parsley sprigs. Enjoy. Refrigerate in an airtight container for up to a day.

Serves 4.

Note: For a variation use the labeneh without the cucumber.

Dessert

Fig Tart With Tahini Cream

Crust

» 2 cups macadamia nuts (or a white nut)
» 2 cups cashews
» ¾ cup raisins, golden
» ¼ tsp. sea salt

In a food processor fitted with an S-blade, combine the ingredients to form a crumbly texture. If using a blender, use the pulse button to combine the ingredients one cup at a time to form a crumbly mixture. Make sure the blender is perfectly dry. Stop the blender to loosen the mixture with a rubber spatula as needed. Pour the loose mixture in a 9-inch tart pan or springform pan lined with parchment paper. Spread the loose mixture out evenly with more content around the rim to form an edge. Then press down with the fingers to form a firm layer of crust.

Note: Any variety of raisin will work for this recipe, but yellow-colored raisins keep this crust a light, golden color. I prefer to use raw macadamia nuts, but if the macadamia nuts are roasted and salted, omit the salt from this recipe.

Filling

» 2½ cups figs (de-stemmed) + ½ cup warm water
» ½ cup honey or liquid sweetener
» 1 Tbsp. carob powder
» ¼ cup coconut oil
» 1 Tbsp. lemon juice
» ¼ tsp. cinnamon

To make the filling, slice the figs in half and soak the figs in water for thirty minutes or longer. Do not drain the water. Using a food processor or blender, combine all the ingredients together until smooth, scraping down the sides of the container with a rubber spatula as needed. Pour into the crust and chill in the refrigerator for four to six hours or in the freezer for two hours or until firm. This dessert stores in an airtight container in the refrigerator up to five days or in the freezer for up to one month. Makes one 9-inch tart.

Tahini Topping

- » 1 Tbsp. white chia seeds + ½ cup water
- » ¾ cup cashews
- » ⅓ cup white sesame seeds (hulled)
- » ½ cup honey or liquid sweetener
- » ⅓ cup coconut oil
- » ¼ cup maple syrup
- » 2 Tbsp. olive oil
- » 1 tsp. ground coriander
- » 1 tsp. vanilla extract
- » Pinch sea salt

Garnish

- » Mint leaves, fresh or dry

Soak the chia seeds for thirty minutes. Soak the cashews and sesame seeds for two hours, and then drain and rinse. Blend all the ingredients together until smooth, scraping down the sides of the blender with a rubber spatula as needed. Served at room temperature, this dessert topping is a sauce. If chilled in the refrigerator for four hours or longer, it becomes a whipped topping. Garnish with mint leaves. Leftover topping can be stored in an airtight container in the refrigerator for up to five days.

Makes over 2 cups topping.

Note: Sesame seeds normally only need one hour soaking, but for this recipe I soaked the sesame seeds and cashews together in a bowl for convenience.

RAW RAW FOR ROMA (ITALIAN)

My memories of Italy were walking on cobblestone pathways, spending time in the coastal ports, and seeing the house where Columbus grew up in Genoa. It's not uncommon for Italian food to be many people's top favorite. Few do pasta better than the Italians. For a fresh version of pasta, I use a spiralizer, or even a vegetable peeler, to make long noodles out of zucchini. It's a wonderful way to replace traditional pasta and cut down on the processed carbs.

Detox Delish

Appetizer

GAZPACHO WITH SOUR CREAM

- » ¼ cup sun-dried tomatoes
- » ½ cup water
- » 2½ cups chopped tomatoes + 1 cup finely diced tomatoes
- » ½ cup chopped cucumbers + ½ cup finely diced cucumbers
- » ½ cup chopped red bell peppers + ½ cup finely diced red bell peppers
- » ¼ cup chopped onions
- » 1 Tbsp. apple cider vinegar
- » 1 Tbsp. olive oil
- » 1 Tbsp. miso
- » ¼ tsp. cayenne (optional or to taste)
- » ¼ tsp. sea salt (optional or to taste)
- » 2 Tbsp. minced cilantro

Garnish
- » 1 avocado, diced
- » ½ cup Cashew Sour Cream (chapter 5)
- » 1 Tbsp. minced cilantro

Soak the sun-dried tomatoes for one hour in ½ cup of water. Do not drain. Setting aside the finely diced produce, blend the chopped produce, sun-dried tomatoes and remaining ingredients until smooth. In a bowl, combine the blended mixture with the finely diced produce. Garnish each serving with diced avocado, a dollop of sour cream, and cilantro. Serve immediately or refrigerate in an airtight container for up to three days.

Serves 4–6.

Side dish

KALE-WALNUT PESTO PASTA

Noodles

- » 4 medium zucchini

To make the noodles, use a spiralizer or vegetable peeler.

Kale-Walnut Pesto

- » 3 cups chopped kale, packed
- » 1 cup walnuts
- » ¼ cup basil leaves
- » ¼ cup nutritional yeast (optional)
- » ½ cup olive oil
- » 2 Tbsp. lime juice
- » 1 clove garlic
- » ½ tsp. sea salt (optional or to taste)

To make the pesto, use a food processor to combine all the ingredients until well combined.

Garnish

- » Basil leaves
- » Cherry tomatoes, halved

Toss the pesto with the zucchini noodles, garnishing the dish with basil leaves and cherry tomatoes. Serve immediately or refrigerate in an airtight container for up to two days.
    Serves 4–6.

Main dish

RAW-SAGNA

Noodles

- » 4 medium zucchini

To prepare the noodles, use a mandoline to slice long strips or finely sliced rounds of peeled zucchini. Set on a paper towel to soak up the juices.

White Nut Ricotta

- » 1 cup almonds
- » 1 cup macadamia nuts
- » 1 cup or more rejuvelac or water
- » 2 Tbsp. lemon juice
- » ¼ tsp. sea salt (optional or to taste)

For a white ricotta, soak the almonds for twenty-four to thirty-six hours, replacing the water every twelve hours.

Pop off the almond skins. Skins can also be removed by blanching the almonds sixty seconds in boiling water and then peeling the skins off. Otherwise, just soak the almonds eight to twelve hours, drain and rinse with the brown skins remaining. Blend all the ingredients together until smooth and pour into a glass jar lined with a nut milk bag or cheesecloth, and let the mixture sit on the counter at room temperature for one to two hours. Lift the contents out of the jar and place in a colander or strainer over a shallow bowl or plate. Place a weight, such as the glass jar just used or a bowl or plate over the contents. Let sit another eight to twelve hours. Drain the excess liquid.

Makes about 2 cups.

Note: The Almond Pulp Ricotta recipe from chapter 5 can be used instead of this recipe. The macadamia nuts do not need soaking.

Tomato Sauce

» 1½ cup sun-dried tomatoes
» ¼ cup dates (honey or medjool), pitted
» ¼ cup water
» 2 Tbsp. lemon juice
» 2 Tbsp. olive oil
» ¼ tsp. sea salt (optional or to taste)

Soak the sun-dried tomatoes and dates in the water for thirty minutes. Using a food processor, combine all the ingredients, include the soaking water for the sun-dried tomatoes and dates.

Makes about 2 cups.

Garnish

» Basil leaves
» Dollop of White Nut Ricotta or Almond Pulp Ricotta
» Cherry tomato halves

Assemble in this order: zucchini slices, ricotta, zucchini slices, tomato sauce, zucchini slices. Garnish with a fresh tomato slice, a dollop of ricotta, and basil leaves. Serve this recipe at room temperature. Or to warm up this raw main dish, place in a food dehydrator for one to two hours at 115 degrees Fahrenheit.

Serves 6–8.

Note: You can also layer in the Kale-Walnut Pesto (above) with the lasagna. If desired, you can also simply buy ricotta.

KALE, CAESAR! (MAIN DISH SALAD OPTION)

Greens

» 1 bunch kale, de-stemmed
» 1 Tbsp. lemon juice
» Pinch of sea salt (optional)
» 1 head romaine lettuce

Thinly slice the kale and massage with the lemon juice and salt until tenderized. Combine with the romaine lettuce.

Dressing

» ⅓ cup cashews
» ¼ cup raisins
» ¾ cup water
» ¼ cup grated fresh horseradish
» 2 Tbsp. dulse flakes
» 2 Tbsp. natural soy sauce
» 2 Tbsp. olive oil
» 2 Tbsp. flax oil
» 2 Tbsp. lemon juice
» 2 Tbsp. miso
» 1 Tbsp. honey or liquid sweetener
» 2–4 cloves garlic
» ½ tsp. wasabi powder or paste
» ½ tsp. sea salt (optional or to taste)

To make the dressing, soak the cashews and raisins in the water for twenty minutes. Do not drain. Blend all the ingredients together until smooth.

Garnish

» Lemon slices
» Ground black pepper (to taste)
» White Nutty Parmesan (recipe below)

Pour half of the dressing in with the greens and keep adding until a desired taste is reached. Garnish with lemon slices and black pepper. Serve with the White Nutty Parmesan. Store this dressing in an airtight container in the refrigerator up to five days.

Serves 4–6.

White Nutty Parmesan

- » 2 Tbsp. golden flaxseed
- » 1 cup macadamia nuts
- » ¼ cup white sesame seeds
- » 2–3 cloves garlic
- » 1 tsp. sea salt (optional or to taste)

In a dry blender, grind the flaxseed to form a flour consistency (if they are not already ground). Pulse the remaining ingredients in the blender one cup at a time until a crumbly texture is formed. Stop the blender to loosen the mixture with a rubber spatula as needed. Mix all ingredients together. Serve immediately or refrigerate in an airtight container up to two weeks.

Makes 2 cups.

Serving suggestion: Add this topping to the pesto, salad, or lasagna.

Note: Macadamia nuts are often salted and harder to find in raw, unsalted form. If this is the case, go much lighter on the salt. Brown flaxseed can be used, but to keep this parmesan white, I went with the golden yellow kind.

Dessert

Ti-raw-misu

Cake

- » 1½ cups almond flour
- » 1½ cups almond pulp (or 1½ cups almond flour)
- » ½ cup cacao powder
- » 2 Tbsp. psyllium husk
- » ⅛ tsp. + pinch sea salt
- » ⅔ cup ripe, mashed avocado (about 1 medium avocado)
- » ½ cup coconut palm nectar or maple syrup

» ½ cup coconut oil, liquefied
» 4 shots espresso (8 oz.)

To make the cake, first combine flour, pulp, cacao powder, psyllium husk, and salt together in a bowl, working the ingredients through the fingers, maintaining a fluffy texture. Add the avocado and continue working the mixture through fingers, keeping the mixture loose. Mix until smooth. Fold in the coconut palm nectar, coconut oil, and espresso. Place contents into a 9 x 9 inch square or round spring form pan lined with parchment paper and dusted with a little cacao powder. Gently press the mixture into one layer; do not pack the layer. Place into the refrigerator or freezer while making the vanilla mousse layer.

Vanilla Mousse

» ½ cup water +1 Tbsp. chia seeds
» ¾ cup cashews
» 2 cups young Thai coconut meat (2–4 coconuts)
» 1¼ cup Probiotic Almond Cream (see chapter 5)
» ⅔ cup honey or liquid sweetener
» ⅔ cup coconut oil, liquefied
» 1 Tbsp. lecithin powder
» 1 Tbsp. psyllium husk
» 1 Tbsp. vanilla extract
» 2 tsp. coffee flavor

Garnish

» 1 tbsp. cacao powder

To make the vanilla mousse, first soak the chia seeds for thirty minutes or overnight in the refrigerator. Soak the cashews for two hours, and then drain and rinse. Then blend the coconut meat, almond cream, honey, soaked chia seeds, and cashews until smooth. With the blender running on low, gradually blend in the coconut oil, lecithin powder, psyllium husk, vanilla extract, and coffee flavor until smooth. Scrape down the sides of the blender with a rubber spatula as needed. Pour the mousse layer into the pan. This is the second layer. To get the air pockets or bubbles out, let sit for ten minutes and then gently lift the pan half an inch off the counter and drop a few times until most of the tiny bubbles pop. Chill in the refrigerator six hours or until firm or in the freezer for two hours or until firm. Using a mesh strainer, dust cacao powder over the top.

Makes one 9 x 9 inch Ti-raw-misu.

Note: If caffeine is one of the ingredients you are eliminating in your diet, but you don't mind a minute amount, you can remove the espresso from the cake and increase the amount of coffee flavor to 2 Tbsp. in the mousse.

HELLO RAW BENTO (JAPANESE)

Growing up in a Japanese American family taught me a love for the sweet and savory flavors of seaweed snacks and an assortment of pickled vegetables such as the daikon radish prepared in this menu. It was my Japanese grandmother, Sue, who always told me to eat more vegetables and fruit. She would also put a miso-mayo spread on baked salmon and vegetables, and I've adopted a slightly fresher version, without the mayo, that browns wonderfully in the food dehydrator just as if baked in the oven.

Appetizer

TAKUAN (DAIKON RADISH)

- » 3 cups thinly sliced daikon radish rounds (or cut in 6-inch strips)
- » 1½ cups warm water
- » 1 Tbsp. sea salt (optional or to taste)
- » ½ cup honey or liquid sweetener
- » ⅓ cup apple cider vinegar
- » 1 tsp. turmeric
- » ¼ tsp. mustard powder
- » ½ tsp. red pepper flakes

In a glass jar, combine all the ingredients and stir until the salt and other ingredients dissolve. Leave on the countertop for eight hours or overnight. Stir again and refrigerate in an airtight container up to one month.

Fills a quart jar.

Note: Takuan is a pickled yellow root made from the daikon radish and is usually made with refined sugar and yellow food coloring. This raw version is a healthy blend of honey and turmeric, which is a natural yellowing color to keep this favorite dish looking traditionally bright and sunny. Takuan is a dish enjoyed with rice or an ingredient inside sushi rolls. This raw version omits boiling and is without the refined, white sugar.

Side dish

MACADAMIA RICE WITH FURIKAKE

Rice

- » ½ cup sesame seeds
- » 5 cups cauliflower, finely diced
- » 2 cups macadamia nuts
- » ¼ cup lemon juice
- » 1 Tbsp. lemon zest
- » 2 Tbsp. olive oil
- » 1 tsp. sesame oil
- » ½ tsp. salt

Soak the sesame seeds for two hours, and then drain and rinse. Place the finely diced cauliflower in a bowl. In a completely dry blender pulse the dry macadamia nuts to form a crumbly texture and add to the bowl. Fold in all other ingredients. Store in an airtight container for up to four days.

Serves 4–6.

Furikake

- » 5 nori sheets
- » ¼ cup sesame seeds, white
- » ¼ cup sesame seeds, black
- » ¼ cup nutritional yeast
- » ¼ tsp. sea salt (optional or to taste)

To make the furikake, break the nori sheets into smaller pieces so they fit into a blender. The blender should be bone dry. Blend the nori until it turns into flakes. Pulse in the remaining ingredients. Store in an airtight container in the refrigerator for up to one month.

Makes about 1 cup.

For each scoop of rice, add one spoon of furikake topping.

Note: You can also try a spoonful of furikake on top of salads, soups, and sandwiches.

Main dish

VEGGIE STEAKS WITH MISO SPREAD

Veggie Steaks

- » 1 large zucchini
- » 1 large eggplant
- » 1 large tomato, firm
- » 1 Tbsp. lemon juice
- » 1 Tbsp. olive oil
- » Pinch sea salt
- » 4–5 sheets of nori seaweed

Slice vegetables into ⅓-inch slices in any shape. Sprinkle with a pinch of salt and rest on a paper towel for twenty minutes to soak up excess juices. Then squeeze lemon juice and drizzle olive oil over the vegetables.

Miso Spread

- » 1 cup cashews
- » ⅔ cup water
- » ½ cup white miso
- » 1 tsp. onion powder
- » ½ tsp. garlic powder
- » ¼ tsp. nutmeg
- » Pinch sea salt

To make the spread, soak the cashews for two hours, then drain and rinse. Blend the cashews and water until smooth. Add in the remaining ingredients. I like to use squeeze bottles to spread the miso topping for a cleaner look. Leftover miso spread can be stored in an airtight container in the refrigerator up to one week.

To assemble the steaks, add a dollop of miso spread and even out over the top of each vegetable slice. Place each vegetable slice directly onto a dehydrator screen tray and warm for four hours at 115 degrees Fahrenheit. As the veggie steaks warm up, excess liquid will come out. Before serving, placed the vegetable steaks onto sheets of nori to soak up the excess juices.

Store up to five days in a sealed container in the refrigerator. To warm, place in the dehydrator thirty minutes to one hour before serving.

Makes 16–22 slices.

Note: My Grandma Sue used to make something like this with miso and mayonnaise on salmon and all sorts of vegetables.

Dessert

JAPANESE MATCHA CHIA PUDDING WITH MANGO

Pudding

- » 3 cups pumpkin yogurt drink (or milk of choice)
- » ⅓ cup + 1 Tbsp. white chia seeds
- » ⅓ cup honey or liquid sweetener
- » 2 Tbsp. coconut oil, liquefied
- » 2 Tbsp. psyllium husk
- » 2 tsp. green tea matcha powder
- » 3–5 drops stevia
- » ½ tsp. green mineral powder (spirulina, chlorella, etc.)
- » Pinch sea salt

Garnish

- » 1½ cups diced mango
- » 2 Tbsp. lemon juice
- » Mint sprigs

In a jar, combine all pudding ingredients and shake for about ten seconds to loosen the chia seeds and psyllium husk. Shake well and pour into serving bowls. Set on the counter twenty minutes, or chill two hours in the refrigerator or even overnight for a thicker consistency. To garnish, combine lemon juice with the diced mango and top each bowl with the fresh mango and mint leaves. Enjoy this dessert chilled, at room temperature, or warmed if desired. Store in the refrigerator in an airtight container up to five days.

Serves 4.

Note: I use white chia seeds for this recipe to make it look more like sago, but the darker chia seeds will work just fine. Psyllium husk is derived from the seeds of the plant Plantago ovata. Chia seeds and psyllium husk are hygroscopic, allowing them to absorb large amounts of liquid.

Health note: Both chia and psyllium husk are high in fiber and work to cleanse the colon.

Muchas G-raw-cias (Mexican)

My first introduction to Mexico was while I was working for the Idaho Department of Agriculture and traveled there to promote Idaho produce. It was in northern Mexico that I had some of the best food in the world, where fresh cream and squeezes of lime seem to be the finishing touch on many dishes.

Appetizer

Chili Con Kraut (dry-salt method)

- » 1 head of red cabbage (about 4–5 lb.)
- » 1 medium onion (about 1 cup)
- » 1 tsp.–1 Tbsp. sea salt (optional or to taste)
- » 1 Tbsp. cumin powder
- » 1 Tbsp. chili powder
- » ½ cup minced cilantro, packed
- » ¼ cup lime juice

With a food processor or by hand, thinly slice the cabbage and onion. Put the slices in a large glass bowl, and then add the salt in with the vegetables. Toss the contents so the salt is spread out evenly. With clean hands, massage and squeeze the contents to release the juices. Add the remaining ingredients. Stuff the vegetables into a glass bowl or glass jar with a weight, ensuring the liquid rises above the vegetables. A little water may need to be added. Cover with a breathable towel and let sit at room temperature and out of direct sunlight for at least three days and up to two weeks or more. Lid and refrigerate for up to two months.

Fills a half-gallon jar.

Note: This appetizer can be eaten immediately after making, but it won't have the fermented aspect without the waiting time.

Side dish

SOUR CREAMED GUACAMOLE

- » 3 medium avocados, ripe
- » 1 cup Cashew Sour Cream (chapter 5)
- » ½ cup finely diced red bell peppers, deseeded
- » 1 Tbsp. lime juice
- » ¼ tsp. cayenne
- » ¼ tsp. garlic powder
- » ¼ tsp. black pepper
- » ¼ tsp. sea salt (optional)

With a fork, mash all the ingredients together until smooth. Serve immediately or refrigerate in an airtight container for up to two days.

Makes about 2 cups.

Note: Serve guacamole with a main dish or cut veggies, or even eat alone.

Health note: Whether eaten or applied directly to the skin, avocados are one of the finest moisturizers with their rich source of healthy fat and phytonutrients.

Main dish

GREEN TACOS WITH GROUND WALNUT

- » 6–8 large romaine leaves
- » 2 Tbsp. flaxseed
- » 2 cups walnuts
- » 1 cup minced mushrooms (button, cremini, shiitake, etc.)
- » ½ cup finely diced red bell peppers

- » 2 Tbsp. minced cilantro
- » 1 Tbsp. apple cider vinegar
- » 1 Tbsp. liquid aminos or natural soy sauce
- » ½ tsp. chili powder
- » ½ tsp. curry powder
- » ½ tsp. onion powder
- » ¼ tsp. garlic powder
- » ¼ tsp. cayenne
- » ¼ tsp. sea salt

For the taco shells, fold the romaine leaves in half so the stem is the base of the taco. If desired, cut each folded leaf so they are 4 inches long.

For the filling, in a dry blender pulse the flaxseed into a flour consistency and set aside in a large bowl. Pulse the walnuts one cup at a time until a crumbly texture is formed, stopping the blender to loosen the mixture with a rubber spatula as needed. Add the crumbled walnut mixture and the remaining ingredients to the bowl with the ground flaxseed and mix well.

To assemble, add about ½ cup ground filling to each lettuce shell. Garnish by adding a dollop of the Sour Cream Guacamole (recipe above). Another option is to pipe it on with a piping bag, a squeeze bottle, or plastic sealed bag with a small incision made at the bottom corner.

Serve immediately or store contents individually for up to three days.

Makes 6–8 tacos.

Note: For a salad option, chop up the bunch of romaine and add the Ground Walnut and Sour Creamed Guacamole on top. Drizzle with 1 Tbsp. lime juice, 1 Tbsp. olive oil, and 1 Tbsp. flaxseed oil, and then toss.

Dessert

VANILLA FLAN WITH SALTED KARMEL

- » ½ cup cashews
- » ½ cup water
- » ¼ tsp. agar powder
- » ½ cup Almond Cream or Almond Yogurt Drink (chapter 5)
- » ½ cup young Thai coconut meat (1 coconut)

- » ¼ cup coconut oil, liquefied
- » 2 Tbsp. honey or a liquid sweetener
- » 2-inch vanilla bean, scraped (or 1 tsp. vanilla extract)
- » ⅛ tsp. orange zest
- » ⅛ tsp. sea salt

Soak cashews for two hours, and then drain and rinse. In a pan, dissolve the agar powder by whisking it with the water. Keep whisking and bring to a boil for one minute. Transfer liquid to a blender. Blend all ingredients together until smooth. Pour filling into six to eight ramekins or small bowls. Chill for two hours or until firm.

Note: Agar powder is not a raw ingredient, but this is primarily a raw-food recipe.

Salted Karmel

- » ⅓ cup maple syrup or coconut palm nectar
- » 1 Tbsp. coconut oil, liquefied
- » 1 tsp. cacao or carob powder
- » ¼ tsp. cinnamon
- » ⅛ tsp. sea salt

To make the topping, place ingredients in a bowl and stir contents together until smooth.

To assemble, add a small spoonful of Salted Karmel to the top of each flan before serving. Refrigerate in an airtight container up to five days.

Serves 6–8.

A Raw-ssian in Moscow (Russian)

My introduction to Russia was watching Russian gymnasts on television during the Olympics; I was fascinated by their stoic strength and grace. I also lived right next to Beijing's Yabaolu, also known as Russiatown, during my time in China. It was my dad who introduced me to the Russian and Ukrainian beet kvass, and a friend of Russian heritage shared with me how her mother made a traditional home favorite of holodetz, a meat jelly I turned into a plant-based dish years later.

Detox Delish

Appetizer

RAW-SSIAN BLACK BREAD CRACKERS

» ½ cup flaxseed + 1 cup water or rejuvelac
» 2 cups leftover nut or seed pulp
» 1 cup ground flaxseed
» 1 cup almond flour or leftover nut or seed pulp
» 2 Tbsp. olive oil
» 2 Tbsp. carob powder or cacao powder
» 2 Tbsp. caraway seed, crushed
» 1 Tbsp. reishi powder (optional)
» 2 Tbsp. honey or liquid sweetener
» 2 tsp. onion powder
» ½ tsp. + ½ tsp. sea salt to sprinkle on top

Soak flaxseed in 1 cup of either water or rejuvelac for two hours. Setting aside ½ tsp. sea salt, combine all ingredients together. Divide the mixture in half to spread ¼-inch thick on two nonstick drying sheets or parchment paper. With a butter knife or bench scraper, score each sheet four times vertically and four times horizontally. Each sheet will have twenty-five crackers. Dehydrate the crackers at 115 degrees Fahrenheit for two hours. Flip the crackers over directly onto a screen tray. Dehydrate for eight to twelve hours or until crisp.

Makes 50 crackers.

Note: I used maple syrup in the recipe because it dries well compared to some other sweeteners.

Side dish

PICKLED RAW BEETS

» 3 cups shredded beets (about 3 medium-size beets)
» ¾ cup apple cider vinegar
» ¾ cup water
» 1 Tbsp. honey or liquid sweetener
» ¼ tsp. sea salt

Put all the ingredients in a jar. Cover the mouth of the jar with a cloth or towel and set on the counter for eight hours out of direct sunlight. Cover the jar and place in the refrigerator for up to five days.

Fills a quart jar.

Main dish

HOLODETZ (RUSSIAN GELLED NON-MEAT VERSION)

» ½ cup thinly sliced mushrooms (button, cremini, shiitake, etc.)
» ⅛ tsp. sea salt
» 1 tsp. natural soy sauce
» ½ cup black olives, sliced in half
» 1 cup water
» ¼ tsp. agar powder
» 1 tsp. miso
» ¾ cup cubed avocado
» Basil

Slice mushrooms and mix with sea salt and natural soy sauce. Set aside for ten minutes. Squeeze out the juice into a bowl and set aside. Set the mushrooms, along with the olives, on a paper towel to get out the juice.

In a pan whisk water and agar powder until dissolved. Then bring to a boil for one minute.

Remove from heat and continue to whisk as it cools. When the liquid is cool enough to touch with a finger, blend or whisk the liquid with the miso and mushroom juice. Place the olives, mushrooms, and avocados in a bowl or Jell-O mold and pour the mixture on top. Set in the refrigerator for two hours or until firm. To remove from the mold, place the mold in hot water for two minutes and flip onto a plate. Garnish with basil and serve with Hot Mustard (recipe below).

Serves 4–6.

Note: Holodetz is a home favorite, traditionally made by boiling pigs feet or the bones of another animal for a few hours. A Ukrainian friend taught me the traditional way to make this years ago, and this vegan version is a tasty comparison.

Note: Agar powder is not a raw product, but it does replace the gelatin from bone marrow from animals as a plant-based replacement. This is traditionally served with hot mustard.

Hot Mustard

- » 1 cup cashews
- » ⅓ cup apple cider vinegar (try with ½ cup)
- » 2 Tbsp. rejuvelac or water
- » 2 tsp. flaxseed, ground
- » 1 tsp. honey or liquid sweetener
- » 1¼ tsp. mustard powder
- » ¼ tsp. horseradish powder (optional)
- » ⅓ tsp. turmeric powder
- » ⅓ tsp. sea salt

Soak cashews for two hours, and then drain and rinse. Blend all the ingredients together until smooth, scraping down the sides of the blender as needed with a rubber spatula. Serve immediately or refrigerate in an airtight container for up to one week.

Makes over 1 cup.

Dessert

Bird's Milk With Chocolate and Raspberries

Filling

- » ¾ cup cashews
- » ⅓ cup water + 1 Tbsp. white chia seeds
- » 2 cups young Thai coconut meat (2–4 coconuts)
- » ¼ cup water
- » ⅔ cup honey or liquid sweetener
- » 1 Tbsp. psyllium husk powder
- » 2 tsp. vanilla extract
- » 2 Tbsp. lecithin powder
- » ¾ cup coconut oil, liquefied
- » ¼ cup cacao butter, liquefied

To make the filling, first soak cashews for two hours, then drain and rinse. Soak the chia seeds in ⅓ cup water for twenty minutes. Blend the coconut meat, cashews, water, and honey until smooth. Scrape down the sides of the blender with a rubber spatula as needed. Blend in the soaked chia seeds, psyllium husk, vanilla extract, and lecithin powder. With the blender running on low, gradually pour in the coconut oil and cacao butter. When blended, pour filling into six to eight small bowls or ramekins and refrigerate for two hours or until firm enough to top with the chocolate sauce.

Chocolate Sauce

» ⅔ cup cacao or carob powder
» ¾ cup maple syrup or liquid sweetener
» ½ cup coconut oil
» ⅓ cup cashews, soaked two hours, rinsed and drained
» ⅛ tsp. sea salt

To make the chocolate sauce, blend all the ingredients together until smooth, scraping down the sides of the blender with a rubber spatula as needed. Add two spoonfuls of chocolate to each mousse filling. Serve the chocolate sauce at room temperature or chilled.

Garnish

» 2 cups raspberries
» 2 Tbsp. lemon juice
» Mint leaves

To make the garnish, add the lemon juice to the raspberries, folding in until all the raspberries are coated. Top each dessert with the raspberries and mint leaves before serving. The Bird's Milk With Chocolate can be stored in an airtight container up to five days.

Serves 6–8.

SEOULFULLY RAW (KOREAN)

My introduction to Korea was a one-semester exchange program at Yonsei University in Seoul, South Korea. I studied the Korean language, and it was only long enough to get some key words, namely menu items.

Korean cuisine is a favorite of mine, and the spicier the better. Kimchee is a Korean staple, and my friends often discussed secret family recipes and the vast array of flavors and techniques used to make it. Even more important are the health benefits of these fermented delicacies.

Fermented vegetables, such as kimchee and krauts, are commonly eaten in small portions and in conjunction with larger meals. The health benefits include improved digestion and immune function. According to author Sandor Ellix Katz, ferments are even known to chelate heavy metals from the body, such as mercury.[1]

Some kimchee recipes often involve heating the paste to dissolve sugar, rice flour, and fish sauce. To keep this recipe naturally uncooked, I used raw honey. Like most cuisines, kimchee seems much saltier in restaurants compared to recipes prepared at home. My friend Mary's mom, Mrs. Han, who is from Korea and living in America, shared that a common water to salt ratio is 6 cups water to 1 cup salt for the kimchee brine. Mrs. Han shared that Korean monks, living on a low sodium diet, prepare their kimchee using a 10 cup water to 1 cup salt ratio. Since I'm on a mission to cut down on salt and get more sodium through whole foods, I created this recipe using even less sea salt but adding plant-based sodium in the form of dulse, a sodium-rich seaweed.

Appetizer

Low-Salt (but sodium-rich) Kimchee (brine method)

Brine

» 12–16 cups water
» ½–1 cup sea salt

Mix the water and salt into a big bowl. Stir the mixture until the salt crystals are dissolved.

Vegetables

» 1–3 heads napa cabbage (about 5 lb.)
» 1 medium daikon radish, shredded (about 2 cups)
» 1 medium carrot, shredded (about 1 cup)

Cut the cabbage crossways into two-inch slices. Place the cabbage in a large bowl with the brine. Put a weight, such as a big plate, on top to submerge the cabbage. Leave for two to four hours, or overnight for a saltier taste. Using a colander, drain the cabbage. Do not rinse. Add the shredded daikon radish and carrots.

Makes half a gallon

Note: When I finish cutting the ruffled leaves to the cabbage stalk, I narrow the cut to 1-inch slices as a personal preference.

Daikon Cube Version of Kimchee

You can make this using primarily daikon radishes instead of cabbage if you prefer. First, use the same brine used above with cubed daikon radishes (5–7 lb.) instead of cabbage. Then make the Red Pepper Mixture below.

Red Pepper Mixture

» 6–8 cloves garlic
» ¼ cup water
» ¼–⅓ cup Korean red pepper flakes
» 2 Tbsp. miso
» 2 Tbsp. honey or liquid sweetener
» 2 Tbsp. kelp powder
» 1-inch cube ginger

To make the Red Pepper Mixture, use a food processor to combine all the ingredients together to form a paste. To omit using a food processor, mince the ginger and garlic as finely as possible and stir in the remaining ingredients until a paste is formed.

To finish the recipe, drain the brine from the vegetables, and then add the Red Pepper Mixture to the vegetables until everything is well coated. Consider wearing gloves, and make sure you don't touch your eyes as you make this. Pack the contents into a glass jar leaving some room at the top. Place the sealed jar in the refrigerator. Store in the refrigerator for up to two months or longer.

Makes half a gallon.

Detox Delish

Side dish

CHAP CHAE

- » 4 medium zucchini
- » 4 cups spinach, packed
- » 3 cups sliced shiitake mushrooms (or button, cremini, etc.)
- » ⅔ cup julienne (matchstick-size) carrots (or Pickled Carrots from chapter 5)
- » ¼ cup onion, julienne sliced
- » ¼ cup natural soy sauce
- » 1 Tbsp. honey
- » 1 Tbsp. white sesame seeds or hemp seed hearts
- » 2 cloves garlic, minced
- » 1½ tsp. sesame oil
- » ¼ tsp. sea salt (optional or to taste)
- » Pinch white pepper

Garnish

- » White sesame seeds or hemp seed hearts

To make the noodles, use a spiralizer or vegetable peeler to slice the zucchini. With the zucchini noodles set aside, combine all other ingredients and let marinate for thirty minutes. Then stir in the noodles. Serve immediately, garnished with sesame seeds or hemp seed hearts, or store in an airtight container for up to two days. For a warm Chap Chae, place contents on one or two nonstick drying sheets and warm in a dehydrator for one to two hours.

Serves 4.

Note: If you are using dried mushrooms, soak in water until they start to plump up. Rinse, drain, and pat with a paper towel.

Main dish

BIBIMBAP

Rice

- » 5 cups cauliflower (2 medium heads or 2 lb.)
- » ⅓ cup sunflower seeds

» ¼ cup sesame seeds
» 1 Tbsp. lemon juice
» 1 Tbsp. olive oil
» 1 tsp. flaxseed oil
» ½ tsp. sesame oil
» ¼ tsp. salt (optional and to taste)

To make the rice, first soak the sesame seeds for two hours, and then drain and rinse. Then chop the cauliflower into small popcorn-size pieces. Combine with the remaining ingredients.

Toppings

Carrot topping

» 1 cup shredded or julienned carrots (or 1 cup Pickled Carrots)
» ¼ tsp. sesame oil
» Pinch sea salt

Spinach topping

» 5 cups spinach, packed
» 1 clove minced garlic
» 1 tsp. honey
» 1 tsp. natural soy sauce
» 1 tsp. olive oil
» Pinch sea salt

Sprouts topping

» 2 cups sprouts (mung beans, broccoli, alfalfa, etc.)
» ¼ tsp. sesame oil
» Pinch sea salt

Zucchini topping

» 2 cups zucchini, halved and thinly sliced
» ½ tsp. honey
» ½ tsp. natural soy sauce
» ¼ tsp. sesame oil
» Pinch white pepper
» Pinch sea salt

Mushroom topping

» 3 cups shiitake mushrooms (or button, cremini, etc.)
» 2 tsp. soy sauce
» 2 tsp. honey
» ½ tsp. grated ginger
» Pinch black pepper
» Pinch sea salt

To prepare the toppings, mix each topping recipe separately. Massage each ingredient to soften the texture, giving it a more tender, cooked feel. Then place each vegetable side by side, but separately, on a nonstick drying sheet or parchment paper and dehydrate at 115 degrees Fahrenheit for three hours.

Note: You may be asking why not just throw all the veggies together and marinate them. Feel free to do that! However, to keep this Bibimbap "Korean style," it is served with each vegetable individually displayed.

Gochujiang Paste

» ¼ cup Korean red pepper flakes
» ¼ cup miso
» 1 Tbsp. honey or liquid sweetener
» 1 Tbsp. olive oil
» 1 Tbsp. water
» 1 clove garlic
» ¼ tsp. sea salt (optional or to taste)

In a bowl mix all ingredients together until a paste is formed. Refrigerate in an airtight container for up to two months.

Note: Because gochujiang preserves well, feel free to double this recipe to have on hand and add to spice up your soups, top salads, or spread on sandwiches. Traditionally it is excellent in Korean lettuce wraps.

To assemble Bibimbap, place the rice at the base of the bowl. For a traditional Bibimbap appearance, place each vegetable topping in a line from the middle of the rice to the outer edge, to form a colorful and circular fan as the topping. Top the middle of the bowl with a dollop of gochujiang paste. Before eating, Koreans will vigorously mix everything together.

Store in an airtight container for up to five days.

Serves 4–6.

Note: Bibimbap can be served in individual bowls rather than one large serving bowl. Bibimbap traditionally is garnished with a raw egg as well as the gochujiang paste. You can use one mango instead of the raw egg, but it is up to you!

Salad option: You can omit the dehydrator and toss all ingredients, the rice, and toppings together in a bowl for a big salad. The gochujiang paste can be added to taste.

Dessert

Su Jung Gwa Dessert Drink

- » 1¾ cups rejuvelac, coconut water, or water
- » 3 Tbsp. maple syrup or liquid sweetener
- » 1 small orange, juiced and zested
- » 4–6 dates (honey or medjool), pitted
- » ¼ tsp. cinnamon
- » 1-inch cube ginger

Garnish

- » 1 Tbsp. pine nuts

Blend the ingredients together and strain through a nut milk bag or sieve. Serve in small bowls or glasses, such as shot glasses. Top each cup with a few pine nuts.

Serves 6–8.

Note: Traditionally this drink is made by boiling all the ingredients together, but this is a fresh approach made without boiling sugar. Su Jung Gwa is a traditional sweet drink enjoyed after a savory Korean meal and is also known to aid in digestion and improve circulation.

CHAPTER 10

Cleansers and Elixirs: It's a Gut Feeling

WHILE RAW-KTAIL ELIXIRS are beverages more for entertaining and Cleansing Tonics for personal detoxification, they can be used interchangeably for benefits, including improved digestion, toxin removal, and energy boosts. They are not to take the place of fresh juices, but some of them provide good sources of hydration throughout the day. Some are quite strong and are enjoyed in smaller doses.

RAW-KTAIL ELIXIRS AND CLEANSING TONICS

ACV QUENCHER

- » 2 cups water
- » 1 Tbsp. apple cider vinegar
- » 2 tsp. liquid sweetener (optional)

Stir and enjoy.

Serves 1–2.

Note: Water can be cool, room temperature, or hot. Apple cider vinegar is a live culture. It is slightly different than a probiotic; it is a prebiotic, which feeds probiotics. This drink improves digestion and increases circulation. Some drink it to control blood sugar levels. If you drink this each day, you can make a gallon-size portion and play around with slightly stronger levels of apple cider vinegar and sweetness to suit your taste.

COLON CLEANSER

- » 2 cups water
- » 2 tsp.–2 Tbsp. bentonite clay

» 1–2 tsp. psyllium husk

Pour contents into a jar with a lid and shake well. Let soak one hour or overnight on the counter so it's ready the next day.

Makes 2 cups.

Note: This is a common routine to clean out the colon, which is a good idea to do before doing a kidney flush or gallbladder flush. Drink this for three to seven days for a good flush, but you can continue for up to two weeks to a month as well. To get the most benefit, do not eat after 5:00 p.m. Around 7:00 p.m. drink up and follow with a glass of water. This whole mixture can be drunk or even split in half to drink over two days. To save time in preparation, double or triple this recipe and drink over a period of a few days. Make sure you are not taking any type of medication during this time. Use distilled water, but you can also use pure water if that's what you have.

FLAME DETOX

This folk remedy is believed to cure the common cold and clear up sinus issues.

» 1 cup horseradish root (about one 7-inch root), peeled and diced
» 1 cup ginger root, diced
» 1 large onion, diced
» 1 orange, sliced
» 1 lemon, sliced
» ½ cup turmeric, diced
» 1 garlic bulb, sliced in half
» 6–8 habanero peppers, de-stemmed and cut in half
» 6 cinnamon sticks
» ¼ cup black peppercorns
» 5 cups apple cider vinegar (raw, unpasteurized)
» ½ cup honey or liquid sweetener (optional or to taste)

Setting the apple cider vinegar and honey aside, place all other ingredients into a half-gallon jar or two pint-size jars, leaving an inch or two of room at the top. Fill the jar with apple cider vinegar until the ingredients are covered. Cap the jar with a non-metal lid. If using a metal lid, place parchment paper between the jar's mouth and lid to prevent corrosion.

Place in a cool place and out of direct sunlight for four to six weeks, giving it a good shake daily (missing a day or two will not hurt it). Next strain the vinegar into a glass jar or bottle. Add honey to taste. Store in the refrigerator up to one year.

Contents fill a half-gallon jar.

Note: This is a potent mixture. Drink 1 Tbsp. or shot glass size in the morning, or whenever you feel like it. I like to offer this to guests just to get a reaction out of them! Add some to water, juice, or even to a salad dressing to spice it up. Due to the acidity of apple cider vinegar, rinse your mouth out with water after drinking to protect your teeth enamel. Some people recommend mixing a little bit of baking soda and water and swooshing it around.

Consider wearing gloves as you make this, and make sure you do not touch your eyes.

LEMON-GINGER-GOJI DETOX

- » 2 cups water
- » ½ lemon, sliced
- » 1 Tbsp. liquid sweetener (optional)
- » 3–5 thin slices of gingerroot
- » 2 tsp. goji berries
- » Dash cinnamon

Place all ingredients except the water in a cup. Heat the water and pour into the cup, almost like a hot tea. Stir and enjoy.

Note: A favorite morning drink of mine, this is a circulation booster. It will also serve as a relaxing evening drink as well. I usually use hot water and steep the ginger for a while, adding the lemon, sweetener, goji berries, and dash cinnamon in very last. This drink served hot is also gentle on a sore throat and can help clear sinus congestion.

RUBY RED KVASS (PROBIOTIC)

Kvass is a Russian and Ukrainian fermented drink. This is an excellent nonalcoholic beverage to serve dinner guests not only as a conversation piece but also for its healing properties as well. It is a blood cleanser and liver detoxifier.[1] My dad got me started on beet kvass. I often enjoy a little bit before going to bed.

» 3½ cups water (or 3 cups water and ½ cup rejuvelac or kvass)
» ½ tsp. sea salt
» 4–6 beets, chopped
» 2 Tbsp. goji berries

In a half-gallon jar add the liquid and salt, stirring until the salt dissolves. Add the remaining ingredients, leaving an inch or two of room at the top of the jar. I recommend you cover this with a lid that is not airtight. This produces a different taste, and covering is optional. (If the lid you have is airtight, open it every few days.) Place in a cool place out of direct sunlight for at least three days and up to one week, agitating the jar daily. After day three, taste daily until the desired tartness is reached. Store in the refrigerator up to two weeks.

You can make three batches with each batch slightly weaker in taste. To start a new batch, strain out the liquid and fill up again with water and salt. Use a ½ cup's worth of kvass from the previous batch as a starter for future batches. Lid and store each batch in the refrigerator up to two weeks.

Makes three batches of a half-gallon jar each.

Note: You may use ⅓ cup pomegranate seeds instead of goji berries. Go Ferment! Lids may be helpful in preventing white mold from growing. If white mold does grow, you can simply scrape it off fully and still drink it, as long as it does not smell or taste off or spoiled.

Fitness and Health

Throughout this book we have looked at how eating healthy can improve health, and eating certain things can help with some health problems. However, staying in motion is also an important part of living light. I stretch and exercise at home as part of my morning routine. I used to be in competitive gymnastics, and although this was years ago, I started lessons again to work on basic moves, improving strength, and flexibility. Walking and dancing are two favorite activities as well. In short, whether basketball, golfing, gardening, or rock climbing, physical activity becomes habit-forming when it's enjoyed.

THE ROLLING STONES: GALLBLADDER FLUSH

The gallbladder is a small sac located right under the liver in the upper right abdomen. Many live without their gallbladder. The gallbladder's main function is to release bile, aiding in digestion and breaking down fats and oils, making them water soluble. Due to the modern diet and environmental toxins, sediments and cholesterol are often too much for the gallbladder to handle. What occurs is sediment buildup and the formation of gallstones, often too big for the body to naturally release. Over time symptoms range from inflammation to pain and discomfort to heartburn and indigestion.

In the fall of 2014 a friend told me about her upcoming surgery for a gallbladder removal. It was shortly after when another friend told me of her experience of a gallbladder flush, where accumulated stones in the gallbladder were released. Believing God has a unique purpose for each organ in the body, it did not take long to decide which camp—gallbladder flush or gallbladder removal—I wanted to be in.

Though I had not had any symptoms of gallbladder problems, I reasoned a good flush was in order simply because I had never done one before. It was Benjamin Franklin who said, "An ounce of prevention is worth a pound of cure."[2] In addition the health benefits of a gallbladder flush promote more energy, cleaner insides, and improved skin.

This is a list of what you need to complete a gallbladder flush:

- 12–20 green apples

- Cold-pressed apple cider

- ¼ cup Epsom salts

- 3 cups water

- ½ cup cold-pressed olive oil, warmed

- 1 grapefruit

- Raw honey (optional)

- Apple smoothie or drink such as ACV Quencher or Flame Detox)

My gallbladder flush takes five to seven days total, with the actual flush being on the second to the last day. Before doing a gallbladder flush, it's a good idea to detox the colon. I recommended a good colon cleanse earlier in this chapter. Do this for at least three days and up to fourteen days before doing a gallbladder cleanse.

Follow the steps below to complete a gallbladder flush:

1. *Preparing your body for the flush:* For the first four to five days, eat 3–5 green apples a day with meals. In between meals drink apple cider or apple juice as well as an apple smoothie or drink. The apples help to soften the gallstones.

2. *Preparing materials for the flush:* On the day of the flush, do not eat any foods with fat. During the day, combine 3 cups water and ¼ cup Epsom salts in a jar. In another jar combine ½ cup olive oil and the juice from one grapefruit.

3. *Complete the flush:* Follow the schedule below to complete the flush.

    2:00 p.m.: Do not consume any food or liquid after this time.

    6:00 p.m.: Drink ¾ cup of the Epsom salt

mixture. If this taste is too bitter, finish the drink with one spoonful honey.

8:00 p.m.: Drink ¾ cup of the Epsom salt mixture. Warm the grapefruit and olive oil by placing the bottled mixture in a pot of warm to hot water.

9:30 p.m.: Visit the bathroom and get completely ready for bed, including brushing your teeth.

9:45 p.m.: Shake the grapefruit juice and olive oil well. While standing up, drink the entire mixture. I use a plastic squeeze bottle, resembling those refillable ketchup bottles in restaurants. This method, or using a straw, will make it much easier to drink.

9:50 p.m.–10:10 p.m.: Immediately after drinking the olive oil and grapefruit juice mixture, lay down on your right side with the right leg drawn up. Be still for at least twenty minutes and try to fall asleep. The gallstones will start to travel down. I've experienced no pain as the Epsom salt mixture opens wide the bile ducts for the stones to pass smoothly.

6:00 a.m.–8:00 a.m.: Drink ¾ cup of the Epsom salt mixture. Rest the entire day.

8:00 a.m.–10:00 a.m.: Drink ¾ cup of the Epsom salt mixture. The flush is underway and several visits to the bathroom will occur as both the colon and the gallbladder release residue and stones.

4. *Transition off the flush:* Drink plenty of water and juices to stay hydrated. Gradually add blended smoothies and soups, along with raw and cooked vegetables. Also, drink a green smoothie with mineral supplements (green or earth minerals) to replenish the minerals in the body.

I've done this flush several times and even on the third flush, I still had stones. Some people need as much as six flushes, with a couple months in between, to get rid of all their stones. Personally I plan to do this flush once or twice a year.

Alternative Gallbladder Flushes

As mentioned, there are many versions of a gallbladder flush. One is to ingest two tablespoons of olive oil followed by a tablespoon of lemon juice on an empty stomach right before bed daily for two weeks.

There is also a gradual gallbladder cleanse. In this cleanse, avoid foods rich in saturated fats and cholesterol, such as meats, eggs, and dairy, for twenty-one days. Increase these foods known to clean the gallbladder: pears, parsnips, turmeric (root or powder), lime, lemons, and seaweeds. Each day, also take two tablespoons of cold-pressed flaxseed oil (some use olive oil, on food or in smoothies).[3] Note, this remedy for clearing up gallstones is also a good way to eat every day to prevent gallstones.

This is my personal story of removing gallstones. The instructions provided are not intended to diagnose, cure, or treat any disease or ailment. Seek advice from a qualified health specialist if you are experiencing gallstone symptoms. Of course, ask them how their gallbladder is. If they don't have their gallbladder anymore, consider getting a second opinion.

Living Food Retreats and Centers

These centers should be helpful for your physical health. However, some of these centers may have spiritual practices that are not Christian and believers may not be comfortable with. Feel free to research these places for yourself.

ANN WIGMORE NATURAL HEALTH INSTITUTE
P.O. Box 429
Rincón, Puerto Rico 00677
(787) 868-6307
Fax: (787) 868-2430
www.annwigmore.org

HALLELUJAH ACRES
916 Cox Road Suite 210
Gastonia, NC 28054
(704) 481-1700
Fax: (704) 481-0345
www.myhdiet.com

HIPPOCRATES HEALTH INSTITUTE & SPA
1466 Hippocrates Way
West Palm Beach, FL 33411
(561) 471-8876
E-mail: info@hippocratesinst.org
www.hippocratesinst.org

OPTIMUM HEALTH INSTITUTE OF AUSTIN
265 Cedar Lane
Cedar Creek, TX 78612
(512) 303-4817
www.optimumhealth.org

Detox Help

These resources include schools, raw food recipe websites, and more that can assist on your journey to detox.

JENNIFER MAC
www.thejennifermac.com
Visit for recipes, tips, and healthy desserts.

LIVING LIGHT CULINARY INSTITUTE
www.rawfoodchef.com
Visit for information about culinary and nutrition programs.

THE DETOX PROJECT
www.detoxproject.org
Visit for testing for chemicals in foods and chemicals
in the body.

INSTITUTE FOR INTEGRATIVE NUTRITION
www.integrativenutrition.com
Visit for information about health coaching and nutrition
curriculum.

RAW FOOD MADE EASY
www.learnrawfood.com
Visit for more raw food recipes.

MATTHEW KENNEY
www.matthewkenneycuisine.com
Visit for information and education about raw food cuisine.

Notes

Introduction

1. "Hippocrates: Quotes," Goodreads, accessed July 23, 2016, https://www.goodreads.com/author/quotes/248774.Hippocrates.

Chapter 1—Green It Like You Mean It

1. Anthony Samsel and Stephanie Seneff, "Glyphosate's Suppression of Cytochrome P450 Enzymes and Amino Acid Biosynthesis by the Gut Microbiome: Pathways to Modern Diseases," *Entropy*, 15 no. 4, (2013) 1416–1463, doi:10.3390/e15041416.
2. "Plato," AZQuotes, accessed July 14, 2016, http://www.azquotes.com/quote/669395.

Chapter 2—Cleansing and Detoxification: A Simple Approach to Good Health and Clean Food

1. Samsel and Seneff, "Glyphosate's Suppression of Cytochrome P450 Enzymes and Amino Acid Biosynthesis by the Gut Microbiome: Pathways to Modern Diseases."
2. Don Huber, interview with author, May 9, 2016.
3. Ibid.
4. There are many foods besides wheat and cane sugar with glyphosate residue, but these two are some of the most common. Non-GMO foods with glyphosate residue have less residue than GMO foods; Huber interview.
5. "IARC Monographs Volume 112: Evaluation of Five Organophosphate Insecticides and Herbicides," International Agency for Research on Cancer, World Health Organization, March 20, 2015, accessed July 15, 2016, https://www.iarc.fr/en/media-centre/iarcnews/pdf/MonographVolume112.pdf.
6. Huber interview.
7. Samsel and Seneff, "Glyphosate's Suppression of Cytochrome P450 Enzymes and Amino Acid Biosynthesis by the Gut Microbiome: Pathways to Modern Diseases."

8. David Wolfe, *Longevity Now: A Comprehensive Approach to Healthy Hormones, Detoxification, Super Immunity, Reversing Calcification, and Total Rejuvenation* (Berkeley, CA: North Atlantic Books, 2013), 157–158.

9. Gabriel Cousens, *Conscious Eating* (Berkeley, CA: North Atlantic Books, 2000), 181–182.

10. Cynthia Ogden, et al., "Prevalence of Childhood and Adult Obesity in the United States, 2011–2012," *Journal of American Medical Association* 311, no. 8 (2014): 806–814.

11. Joel Fuhrman, *Eat to Live: The Amazing Nutrient-Rich Program for Fast and Sustained Weight Loss, Revised Edition* (New York: Hachette Book Group, 2011), 18.

12. Ibid., 157–158.

13. "Albert Einstein Quotes," BrainyQuote, accessed July 15, 2016, http://www.brainyquote.com/quotes/quotes/a/alberteins133991.html.

14. Fuhrman, *Eat to Live*, 17.

15. Don Colbert, *Toxic Relief: Restore Health and Energy Through Fasting and Detoxification* (Lake Mary, FL: Siloam, 2003), 15.

16. David Wolfe, *Longevity Now*, 157.

17. William Davis, *Wheat Belly: Lose the Wheat, Lose the Weight, and Find Your Path Back to Health* (New York: Rodale, 2011), 16–18.

18. Ibid.

19. Anthony Samsel and Stephanie Seneff, "Glyphosate, Pathways to Modern Diseases II: Celiac Sprue and Gluten Intolerance," *Interdisciplinary Toxicology* 6, no. 4 (2013): 159–184, accessed July 18, 2016, http://www.ncbi.nlm.nih.gov/pmc/articles/PMC3945755/.

20. William Davis, *Wheat Belly Total Health: The Ultimate Grain-Free Health and Weight-Loss Life Plan* (New York: Rodale, 2014).

21. Samsel and Seneff, "Glyphosate, Pathways to Modern Diseases II: Celiac Sprue and Gluten Intolerance."

22. Mark Hyman, *The Blood Sugar Solution: 10-Day Detox Diet* (New York: Little, Brown and Company, 2014), 113–115.

23. Huber interview.

24. Samsel and Seneff, "Glyphosate, Pathways to Modern Diseases II: Celiac Sprue and Gluten Intolerance."

25. "IARC Monographs Volume 112: Evaluation of Five Organophosphate Insecticides and Herbicides."

26. Paul Pitchford, *Healing With Whole Foods: Asian Traditions and Modern Nutrition* (Berkeley, CA: North Atlantic Books, 1993), 382.

27. Fuhrman, *Eat to Live*, 152–153.

28. Ibid., 158, 309.

29. Colbert, *Toxic Relief*, 79.

30. Wolfe, *Longevity Now*, 165.

CHAPTER 3—THE FAST AND THE CURIOUS: THE BENEFITS OF FASTING

1. Books that talk about daily fasting include *Quantum Eating: The Ultimate Elixir of Youth* by Tonya Zavasta.

2. Fuhrman, *Eat to Live*, 307.

CHAPTER 4—RAW FOOD BASICS: SHOPPING LIST AND TIPS

1. "Dirty Dozen: EWG's 2015 Shopper's Guide to Pesticides in Produce," Environmental Working Group, accessed July 20, 2016, http://www.ewg.org/foodnews/dirty_dozen_list.php.

2. A small amount of papaya available in the United States is GE. If you want to avoid GE foods, buy organic.

3. A small amount of sweet corn available in the United States is GE. If you want to avoid GE foods, buy organic.

4. "Clean Fifteen: EWG's 2015 Shopper's Guide to Pesticides in Produce," Environmental Working Group, accessed July 20, 2016, https://www.ewg.org/foodnews/clean_fifteen_list.php.

5. Fuhrman, *Eat to Live*, 305.

6. Wolfe, *Longevity Now*, 163.

7. Tonya Zavasta, *Your Right to Be Beautiful: The Miracle of Raw Foods* (Cordova, TN: BR Publishing, 2003), 126–127.

8. Colbert, *Toxic Relief*, 16–17.

9. Wolfe, *Longevity Now*, 154.

10. Ibid.

CHAPTER 5—FERMENTATION AND PROBIOTICS: IT'S ALIVE!

1. Sandor Ellix Katz, *The Art of Fermentation: An In-Depth Exploration of Essential Concepts and Processes From Around the World* (White River Junction, VT: Chelsea Green Publishing, 2012), 97.
2. Ann Wigmore, *The Hippocrates Diet and Health Program: A Natural Diet and Health Program for Weight Control, Disease Prevention, and Life Extension* (Pennington, NJ: Avery, 1984), 52–53.
3. Cousens, *Conscious Eating*, 485–486.
4. Katz, *The Art of Fermentation*, 31.
5. Ibid., 26.
6. Ibid., 99.
7. Ibid., 98–106.
8. Wigmore, *The Hippocrates Diet and Health Program*.
9. Katz, *The Art of Fermentation*, 185.

CHAPTER 6—GET JUICED: FROM PULP FICTION TO PULP KITCHEN

1. Colbert, *Toxic Relief,* 64.
2. Charlotte Gerson and Morton Walker, *The Gerson Therapy: The Proven Nutritional Program for Cancer and Other Illnesses* (New York: Kensington Publishing Corp, 2006).
3. Ibid., 119–122.
4. Pitchford, *Healing With Whole Foods*, 537–538.
5. Ibid., 329.
6. Jay Kordich, *The Juiceman's Power of Juicing* (New York: William Morrow & Company, 1992), 30, 178.
7. Ibid., 30, 192
8. Pitchford, *Healing With Whole Foods*, 617.
9. Ibid., 622.
10. Ibid., 20.
11. Ibid., 537.
12. Kordich, *The Juiceman's Power of Juicing*, 195.
13. Pitchford, *Healing With Whole Foods*, 544.
14. Ibid.
15. Ibid., 622.

16. Ibid., 616–617.
17. Ibid., 538.
18. Ibid., 558.
19. Katz, *The Art of Fermentation*, 136.

CHAPTER 9—RAW CUISINE AROUND THE WORLD
1. Katz, *The Art of Fermentation*.

CHAPTER 10—CLEANSERS AND ELIXIRS: IT'S A GUT FEELING

1. Katz, *The Art of Fermentation*, 136.
2. "Benjamin Franklin: Quotes," Goodreads, accessed July 25, 2016, http://www.goodreads.com/quotes/247269-an-ounce-of-prevention-is-worth-a-pound-of-cure.
3. Pitchford, *Healing With Whole Foods*, 323.

the JENNIFER MAC™

CUISINE | HEALTH | BEAUTY

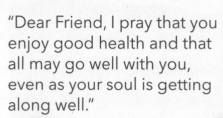

"Dear Friend, I pray that you enjoy good health and that all may go well with you, even as your soul is getting along well."

3 John 1:2

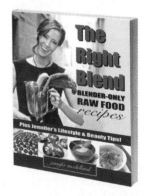

Jennifer Mac is the author of *The Right Blend: Blender-only Raw Food Recipes* and shares her delicious recipes, health-promoting lifestyle, and natural beauty tips. Jennifer Mac's passion is to share with others how to *be deliciously healthy®* using real foods and real ingredients from her home to yours. Growing up on a farm in Idaho, Jennifer Mac got her start pioneering the raw food movement in China after becoming a chef from Living Light Culinary Institute in Northern California.

Visit her website, TheJenniferMac.com. Don't start perfect, just start. Join Jennifer Mac.

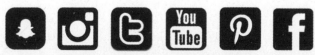

@TheJenniferMac

CONNECT WITH US!

CHARISMA HOUSE

(Spiritual Growth)

f Facebook.com/CharismaHouse

🐦 @CharismaHouse

📷 Instagram.com/CharismaHouseBooks

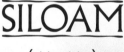

SILOAM

(Health)

📌 Pinterest.com/CharismaHouse

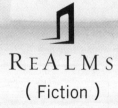

REALMS

(Fiction)

f Facebook.com/RealmsFiction

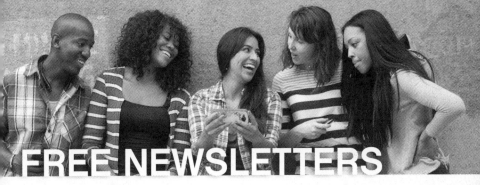